Contents

Preface   iv

1 Some background information   i

2 Problems of morale   5

3 The junior school age   14

4 A fresh start for the older child   29

5 Word-endings and word-beginnings   34

6 Arithmetic   51

   Appendix

       Section I   Consonants for recognition   58
       Section II   More vowel sounds   60
       Section III   Single and double consonants in the
                     middle of a word   63
       Section IV   Word-endings   64
       Section V   groups D and F of Section IV   69

   References   71

   Index   73

Preface

This book is a supplement to *On helping the dyslexic child**, and we suggest that readers should use the two books in combination.

Basic information designed to show what dyslexia is — or, more strictly, how a dyslexic child can be recognised — is contained in the earlier book and is not repeated here. Since *On helping the dyslexic child* was first written, however, demands for assessment and teaching have grown in a quite remarkable way, and as a result we have had the chance to study many more dyslexic children of all ages. We have also had the chance to exchange ideas with about a dozen part-time teachers who work in collaboration with the University Department of Psychology at Bangor and who have been making a special study, each in a one-to-one relationship, of the needs of dyslexic children. On the basis of this later experience we have decided that there are various ways in which *On helping the dyslexic child* required supplementation. There are few suggestions, for instance, on how to adapt our systematic phonic programme to the needs of younger children, i.e. those in the 8-9 age range; nothing is said about the teaching of arithmetic or handwriting, although problems often arise in both these areas, and little help was given on the question of how to guide older pupils, aged 14-15 and upwards, into more advanced spelling after the elementary stages had been covered. These gaps we are now attempting to fill.

Although we have made a number of cross-references to *On helping the dyslexic child* in this present book, we have not made any detailed suggestions as to how exactly the two books should be combined. This is something which we feel should be left to the judgement of the teacher.

---

*   Written by T. R. Miles and published in 1970 by Methuen Educational Ltd.

We should like to emphasise, however, that neither book is a *sequel* to the other. Our suggestion is not that a teacher should finish the one and then proceed to the other; it is rather that he should move from one to the other in accordance with the child's needs. For example, if you are teaching a dyslexic child of seven or eight, the material on pp. 14-23 of this book and in Section I of the Appendix will with almost certainly what you need at the start. Then, when you are satisfied that the child can successfully match particular sounds with particular letters or combinations of letters, you will probably want to pass on to the word-lists and exercises contained in *On helping the dyslexic child*. If the child shows uncertainty as to whether to put *k* or *ck* in a particular word, this is the right time to tell him the rule given on p. 29 of this book, while if you are doing words such as *rattle* and *matter* which are given on p. 49 of *On helping the dyslexic child,* this may well be the right time to introduce the rule, given on p. 28 of this book, that when a short vowel sound is required the consonant which follows should be doubled. The main requirement is that the child should not be expected to spell a word until he has been introduced to the rules which tell him how to set about doing so. To requiie him simply to 'remember' the spelling of long words is to fail to understand the problem.

We should like to take this opportunity of expressing our gratitude to the many people with whom we have exchanged ideas on dyslexia in recent years, including, not least, those parents and children who have visited Bangor and have made clear to us what dyslexic difficulties involve. In this connection we should like to single out for special mention the two Christophers, both themselves dyslexic, one of whom contributed the account of his personal difficulties on p. 13, the other the writing patterns on p. 19.

We are also very grateful to the members of the Bangor team of teachers for the many helpful ideas which they have provided. In particular we should like to thank the late Aline Wiggin, formerly of St Mary's College, Bangor; Chapter 3 reflects her influence in all kinds of ways, and the section of handwriting (pp. 18-21) is based almost entirely on material supplied by her. We should also like to thank Eileen Stirling and Cecily Garratt for their help with Chapter 3 and Chapter 5. Finally we should like to express special gratitude to Alun Waddon, lecturer in the Department of Psychology, who has given many hours to the assessment and teaching of dyslexic children and from whose suggestions we have profited in all kinds of ways.

Bangor, 1973   T R M

E M

CHAPTER ONE

Some background information

One of the main objectives in the early chapters of *On helping the dyslexic child* was to describe the ways in which dyslexic children are different. The central theme was this: if a child of ordinary ability is late at learning to read and has special difficulty over spelling, and if, in addition, he shows confusion over getting things into the right spatial and temporal order, one should regard him as having a distinctive disability requiring special attention. If the argument in *On helping the dyslexic child* is correct, it is wrong – and indeed, irresponsible – to say to parents 'Don't worry; he'll grow out of it'. On the contrary it is essential that special remedial teaching should be provided immediately by someone who knows what the difficulties are. Simply correcting the child's mistakes and relying on constant repetition is unlikely to be effective and may well give rise to increasing frustration and all-round loss of confidence.

The commonly accepted name for this disability (or group of disabilities) is *dyslexia*. Other words have been used in the past, for example *word-blindness, strephosymbolia* (literally 'turning of symbols'), *developmental aphasia, specific developmental dyslexia,* and *specific language disability*. Some of these terms may not be very elegant, but there can be little doubt as to the kinds of difficulty to which they refer.

Since, however, some parents and teachers may still hear hostile remarks about dyslexia and even meet those who profess 'not to believe in it' (though one hopes they are a dwindling number), it seemed to us that it might be helpful to give some information on the historical side and to follow this up with an account of some of the things which are now being done in Great Britain in the attempt to make dyslexia more widely recognised. It is to be hoped that such information will contribute to removing some of the unnecessary bickering which perhaps surprisingly — still seems to persist when the problems of the dyslexic child are discussed.

One of the early pioneers who described this condition was a Glaswegian doctor, James Hinshelwood. He used the term *word-blindness*. His suggestion was not, of course, that these children were blind in any literal sense but rather that they were 'blind' to the *look* of the words which they needed to read and write; printed or written words were simply marks on paper, not conveyers of meaning. Hinshelwood was convinced — correctly, as it now seems — that their disabilities were due to some kind of failure of development in the nervous system, and he made a passionate plea (which seems to have been completely ignored) that their problems should be taken seriously. Details of his two important books, published in 1900 and 1917, are given in references 7 and 8, page 71.

Another pioneer was the American psychiatrist, S.T. Orton, whose book, *Reading, Writing and Speech Problems in Children* (reference 10, p. 71) was published in 1937. Orton noticed that some children seemed to find it easier to write from right to left rather than the other way round and that sometimes letters or diagrams were reproduced mirror-wise. This condition, which he called *strephosymbolia* (literally 'turning of symbols'), was due in his opinion to some abnormality of brain function; he shared with Hinshelwood the view that the difficulties were constitutional in origin. As a psychiatrist he was clearly very much aware of the frustration and uncertainty to which these children were exposed. The Orton Society, called after him, is now a thriving concern, and methods of teaching based on his original insights have been carefully worked out by Anna Gillingham and Bessie Stillman (see reference 3, p. 71).

Some interesting work was done in Scotland before the Second World War by M. MacMeeken (reference 9, p. 71). MacMeeken's research involved taking 392 children (ages $7\frac{1}{2}$–$10\frac{1}{2}$ years) and picking out for special study those whose reading attainment lagged appreciably behind their intellectual level as judged by a traditional intelligence test. She regarded their difficulties as having two main characteristics. 'For these children . . . . .', she writes, 'no word exists to be recognised until the child has rendered his written symbol in terms of the spoken word' (op.cit., p. 47). Secondly, 'the whole syndrome is one of serious directional confusion' (ibid. p. 47). She concludes that 'quite definitely . . .

the difficulties are aphasic in character' (ibid. pp. 47-48). This analogy with mistakes made by adult aphasic patients (i.e. those whose thought and speech have been disturbed by brain injury) seems to us an important insight. It does not, of course, follow that children with the dyslexic group of disabilities can be described as brain-*damaged;* one should perhaps think rather in terms of failure of development. MacMeeken's evidence, however, gives clear support to the view that the difficulties are constitutional in origin and are not the result of poor teaching or of too much pressure by over-anxious parents.

In general, however, as far as Great Britain is concerned, the needs of the dyslexic child do not seem to have been at all widely recognised in the 1940s and 1950s; and as late as 1959, at a conference of educational psychologists held at Nottingham, few speakers came out with any strong support for the idea that some children could be described as *dyslexic.* (It is possible that some of those present mistakenly supposed that such a description implied that nothing could be done; and indeed it seems likely that at least part of the controversy about the value of the term dyslexia has arisen as a result of misunderstanding rather than genuine disagreement.) In 1962, the Invalid Children's Aid Association, under its Chairman, Dr Alfred White Franklin, convened a meeting at St Bartholomew's Hospital in London, at which, despite some hostility, the problems of the dyslexic child were squarely faced. The result of this meeting was the setting up of the Word-Blind Centre in London, where the attempt was made to combine both teaching and research: practical help was given to selected children who displayed the dyslexic group of symptoms, while data were systematically collected and analysed with a view to finding out more about these children and discovering how they differed from their non-dyslexic contemporaries. The results of this research have been published by Sandhya Naidoo (see reference 5, p. 71), and, amongst other interesting findings, she concluded that the learning failure on the part of her dyslexic children was 'not primarily the result of deficient educational opportunity or of severe emotional disturbance' (op.cit., p. 109), but that, on the contrary, 'some reading and spelling disorders are constitutionally determined' (ibid. p. 114).

Another interesting development has been the formation of local Dyslexia Associations. Their main purpose has been to try to persuade Local Authorities to do more to meet the needs of dyslexic children

3

and to prevent the more gross cases of mishandling. Many of the members of these Associations were in fact parents of dyslexic children; and they no doubt felt that more would be achieved if they acted as members of an Association rather than as individuals. At the time of writing a British Dyslexia Association has just been formed, and there seems every hope that it will be influential. Parents of dyslexic children may therefore be considerably helped if they establish contact either with their local Dyslexia Association or with the British Dyslexia Association (present address, 18, The Circus, Bath).

In 1970 there was official recognition of dyslexia by Parliament. In the *Chronically Sick and Disabled Persons Act* of that year there is a reference to those with 'acute dyslexia', and it is now mandatory upon Local Education Authorities to furnish information about them. (The word 'acute' is perhaps unfortunate, since this implies the sudden onset of a disability; but all the literature, as well as the brochures issued by local Associations and others, make clear the kind of disabilities which are intended.) Later a committee was set up under the Chairmanship of Professor J. Tizard to advise the Minister of State for Education, Mrs Thatcher, on what needed to be done. The Tizard Report, published in 1972, was something of a dissapointment to local Associations, since it appeared to be discussing poor reading and spelling in general, not the special needs of the dyslexic child. It does, however, contain a number of humane recommendations, e.g. that more provision should be made for the teaching of reading and spelling and that those with difficulties in this area should receive special consideration in examinations.

In the present climate of opinion, therefore, it is still not impossible that parents who believe their child to be dyslexic may be bewildered by contradictory advice. If the disputes were simply over a name, that is to say, if all those concerned were in agreement as to what should be done and differed only the question of what word best described the condition, there would be little cause for concern. Our experience suggests, however, that often those who do not like to use the word *dyslexia* (or some equivalent word) are those who fail to appreciate the child's needs. To say that he is dyslexic implies that he has a disability and that special teaching will be required if he is to compensate for it; the word *dyslexia* invites us to take the disability *seriously*. Moreover, since the mistakes made by the child are manifestations of this disability, it is wrong to dub him as 'careless' or 'lazy' or to regard his parents as

4

'neurotic' if they press for adequate teaching facilities. Much more is involved, therefore, than a dispute over what word to use; and if parents find themselves involved in controversy as to whether such a thing as dyslexia exists at all, our suggestion is that they should make sure that their child is in the hands of someone who genuinely understands his difficulties.

We are not claiming that there is a single set of symptoms which characterises all dyslexic children or that there is one single type of brain failure which causes these symptoms. We have in fact met a variety of difficulties: some dyslexic children are clumsy, some are not; some continue to reverse *b*s and *d*s up to age twelve or beyond whereas some grow out of it much earlier; in some cases the difficulty seriously affects performance in arithmetic, while in other cases it does not; some have difficulty in grasping what a rhyme is; some have difficulty in repeating polysyllabic words, and so on. It is most unlikely that all the symptoms will be present in any one child, and it may even be the case that he displays difficulties (e.g. *b-d* confusion) on some occasions and not on others. It is perhaps appropriate, therefore, to regard dyslexia as a family or cluster of disabilities rather than as a single condition. The important point is that the children who have these disabilities need help.

CHAPTER TWO

Problems of morale

By the time a dyslexic child reaches the age of about ten he will already have a long history of failure behind him, and this is likely to be all the more painful if his difficulties have not been understood. It therefore seems important to ask, What does this failure *mean* to him?

We can perhaps reconstruct his earlier experience somewhat as follows. One of the things which happened when he first went to school

5

was that his teacher put various chalk-marks on the blackboard. Like others in the class he may perhaps have been able to learn the names of individual letters and numerals, but once the combinations of letters reached a certain degree of complexity he found himself not knowing what to do. Other children in the class were responding in such a way that they gained the teacher's approval. He, too, could gain the teacher's approval if questions were oral, but if he was required to make the right noise when a complex group of letters was put before him, or carry out a complex set of movements with his pencil when words were said to him, the result was almost always complete failure. Small wonder if he felt utterly bewildered!

If a child has an obvious disability, for example if he is lame or paralysed, both he and the adults at least know what to expect. Even in the case of a child who is slow at learning and is put in a special class, the problem is manageable and clear. For a dyslexic child, however, unless his dyslexia is recognised, there must always be the nagging uncertainty, 'Am I stupid? Am I mad? Why am I different from the others?' Vague, unformulated fears are perhaps even more unpleasant than a clearly recognised disability; and in this connection we should like to quote what seems to us to be a really telling sentence from *The Pirate,* by Sir Walter Scott: 'The most cruel wounds are those that make no outward show'. In view of what they have been up against, it is remarkable that so many dyslexic children are as resilient and happy as they are.

How, then, can a teacher help to build confidence in a dyslexic child? The first requirement, in our view, is that he should continually make clear that he understands what the child finds difficult, or, if he is new to the task, that he will *try* to understand. This means, for instance, that he will not show surprise if a word which has been spelled correctly is misspelled immediately afterwards; he will not simply regard the child as 'careless' if he leaves parts of a word out, or as 'lazy' or 'lacking in keenness' if he tires easily. At all ages the amount of effort required from a dyslexic child to produce a particular result is much greater than would be required from a non-dyslexic child, and if a teacher fails to appreciate this it is hard to see how a really understanding relationship between him and the child can ever be possible.

This does not mean, of course, that one should simply hand out indiscriminate praise. Like anyone else, the dyslexic child has his self-respect, and none of us likes to be told we have done well when this is blatantly not the case; indeed this kind of deception is easily seen through. There was a highly intelligent ten-year-old whom one of us saw recently whose father had congratulated him on a slightly improved result in a spelling test at school. According to his father, the boy had replied in a puzzled way, 'But I've got a lot of them wrong'. The problem for the teacher is often that of finding what is the appropriate standard to expect. Thus it seems perfectly correct to say to a dyslexic child, 'Yes, I agree you have made some mistakes. But I still say you have done well; it is an improvement on last week and, in view of your disability, it is a satisfactory result'. If, on the other hand, there is no improvement, one is not being much of a friend if one tries to pretend that there is. The response should perhaps be: 'Yes, such-and-such still seem to be causing you difficulty; let us see if we can explore some different way of helping you'.

In Bangor we have always made clear to the child from the outset that he is dyslexic. This does not, of course, mean that we necessarily fire the actual word 'dyslexia' at, say, an eight-year-old. We do, however, make it clear that he has a disability; we explain that he is not stupid but that there are some things — particularly to do with spelling and reading — which he may find more difficult than do other boys and girls in the class. The actual name of the disability can be mentioned whenever it seems appropriate, provided only that one has first specified the kinds of thing which the child can expect to find difficult.

We then try to help him to learn from experience where his limitations lie. He needs to know, for instance, that he may take longer than other children in the class to read the same amount of material, that he is less likely than they are to remember correct spellings several days later, and that those with his disability often find difficulty in learning arithmetical tables. On the other hand, it is perfectly possible for him, once he has been shown how to do a word belonging to a particular group, to do other words in that group; thus if he has been shown *gate* he can be expected — at least in that context — to be able to spell *date*. It is very discouraging, however, if time after time he is told that his answer is 'wrong' by someone who has no clear understanding of what can reasonably be expected of him. If he is doing free composition, it is wise to make clear to him that for this particular purpose mistakes in spelling do not matter (compare p. 26); if he is receiving special coaching in spelling, we suggest that, as far as possible, *he should not be given the chance* to spell words wrongly. Thus it would be wrong to give him the word *ground* until one knows that he can operate with the double consonants *gr* and *nd* and is able to represent the *ou* sound. If there is any doubt one should go back and revise these earlier procedures first; they are, as it were, the 'components' of spelling the word *ground,* and it is misguided to expect him to give you the final product when he cannot give you the parts from which it is made up. It is better that he should attempt an easier task and have the satisfaction of success rather than attempt a more complex task before he is ready for it and have the frustration of failure.

From the teacher's point of view one of the important skills is the ability to 'read the signs' – to recognise what kinds of thing the child finds difficult and why – and to adapt accordingly. Often this means slowing down and not attempting to do too much too soon. Being 'kind' to a dyslexic child without understanding his difficulties is insufficient if you are trying to teach him to read and spell; and, indeed, if you do not know what to expect, the sorts of mistake which he may make will be so exasperating to you and bewildering to him that even being kind will not be easy.

We should next like to call attention to some of the more subtle ways in which dyslexic disabilities affect the child's life. We shall be considering in Chapter 3 some of the incidental effects of his failure to learn to read easily (see p. 14). Here we shall mention some of the possible effects if he has difficulties in orientation and sequencing.

We have continually met dyslexic children who cannot easily arrange material in the right order. Many, for instance, find it hard to repeat the months of the year correctly, and almost all find it hard to say them backwards. (A few even have difficulty with days of the week, though this is less common, perhaps because the task is shorter or, possibly, more familiar). Even those who in other respects are obviously intelligent may be unable to say what month it is or give the month and year of their birth. Several are reported to have shown confusion over *time* words, e.g. by using 'yesterday' when they meant 'tomorrow'; and one older boy, according to his parents, did not always seem to know the correct day of the week or time of day; thus he might announce that he was 'off to the shops', either forgetting that it was a Sunday or not noticing that it was 7.30 in the evening when all shops would be shut.

Not all dyslexic children make such mistakes, but it seems important that parents and teachers should be alerted to this kind of possibility. One cannot help wondering if an insecure sense of time makes it impossible for some dyslexic children to 'look forward' to things, e.g. to Christmas or to their birthday. Difficulty with arithmetic is perhaps part of the same handicap. To work out for oneself that it is eighteen days to Christmas one has not only to know that it is now December 7th and that Christmas Day is December 25th; one has also to be able to subtract seven from twenty-five. It may therefore help a dyslexic child if he is shown how a calendar works or if he is told that a particular event will take place soon or in a few weeks. One cannot take for granted that he has learned this kind of thing for himself.

Finally, we should like to comment on some of the ways in which the presence of someone with dyslexia affects social relationships both within the family and at the child's school.

As regards relationships within the family, it is remarkable, in our experience, how successful most families have been in dealing with potential sources of stress. We have admittedly had evidence of behaviour problems which occurred *before the dyslexia was recognised* – the boy who slammed the door in rage because he had been misunderstood, the girl who played truant for a time, etc. Once the fact of dyslexia is acknowledged, however, our experience is that most parents find themselves able to be tolerant and that most children feel under very much less strain.

There may, of course, be extra problems if an older child is dyslexic while his younger brother or sister is not; it is not surprising if the dyslexic child feels a certain reluctance to accept help! Our experience suggests that full and frank discussion is the most appropriate answer. As usual, it is misunderstanding which seems to create the problems, and if everyone knows what kinds of thing a dyslexic child finds difficult a major cause of unhappiness is removed.

We have, however, been concerned to note the *unnecessary* strain to which parents of dyslexic children have sometimes been exposed. The tradition, alas!, seems to die hard in educational circles that, where something has gone wrong on the social side, 'it is all the parents' fault';

and we have found that, time and time again, parents of dyslexic children have been told — or at least allowed to believe — that their own anxiety was the main cause of the child's difficulties. (Such 'experts' often seem reluctant to consider even the possibility that the child is suffering from a constitutional disability; and it seems hard to understand why such alleged anxieties should result in failure at specific tests, such as reading, spelling, saying numbers backwards, etc., and should not extend e.g. to oral work or to art.) Three examples from our experience must suffice. In one case the father of a bright dyslexic boy of ten was asked by an educational organiser, 'What have you *done* to the boy to make him like this?' In another case the mother of an exceptionally bright dyslexic boy of thirteen had parted from her husband; not surprisingly she was made to feel that the boy's difficulties were the direct result of the disruption of the home. Thirdly, there was the case of a woman who had adopted three boys but who was herself unmarried. One of these boys, though bright, was in fact found at age nineteen to be severely dyslexic, with a special weakness at tasks involving short-term memory. Time and time again this woman had been led to believe that absence of a father was the main causal factor (this, despite the fact that this absence had *failed* to produce dyslexia in two of her three sons!). Such handling seems to us to constitute downright unkindness, and it therefore seems important that parents should be reassured, if they have received such criticism, not to take it seriously.

Parents of dyslexic children are also accused sometimes of being 'over-protective'. Here, again, it seems to us desirable that they should use their own judgement as to what the child needs rather than be put off by what others think he ought to need. We have regularly found that a dyslexic child may be two years, or even more, behindhand when it comes to taking examinations such as C.S.E. and O level. We also have reason to suppose that in some cases dyslexia can hold back general emotional maturity. Thus it may well be — at least in these cases — that a dyslexic child is in need of a certain amount of extra 'mothering'; and we very much hope that fear of seeming to be what is unkindly called in some circles an 'anxious mum' will not prevent mothers from giving a dyslexic child the attention which they can see is necessary.

It is sometimes implied that the notion of dyslexia is an invention by over-ambitious middle-class parents who cannot accept the fact that their child is none too bright and wish to make some further excuse for his failure in school. Our experience does not bear this out. We have in fact met few cases where the parents believed their child to be dyslexic and were mistaken, though occasionally we have met cases where the child's other needs (e.g. for psychiatric help) were more pressing. We have, however, met plenty of cases where the child was in fact dyslexic but where the parents made clear that, if the child was found simply to be rather slow, this would not distress them unduly. Sneers that dyslexia is a middle-class invention are unkind and unjustified.

Another piece of educational folk-lore which seems to need challenging is the view that parents should never attempt to teach their own children. In some cases, it is true, families may prefer that the teaching should be done by a person outside who has had previous experience of dyslexia. If no such person is available, however, it seems to us perfectly reasonable that parents should learn to undertake the job themselves. On several occasions we have in fact invited mothers (and on one occasion a father) to sit in for a week while the child received daily lessons from our own teachers, and we have then encouraged them to take over the teaching. We do not wish to minimise the amount of patience and skill which this arrangement calls for, nor to press parents into such an arrangement against their better judgement. It is important, however, that they should not be discouraged from the attempt simply because 'experts' have led them to doubt their own competence.

We are sometimes asked what are the long-term prospects for a dyslexic child. It is difficult to answer with any high degree of assurance. We are in no doubt that it is possible for those with dyslexia to achieve considerable success in academic or other fields, since we have met people who have done so. Passing examinations may take longer, and quite a number of adults with residual dyslexic signs have reported to us that they are still poor spellers and (in some cases) slow readers. It seems likely, therefore, that the difficulties do not disappear completely, but our experience suggests that they can be largely compensated for and are unlikely to cause permanent unhappiness. Our general feeling is that a dyslexic child should be allowed to go at his own pace and that parents should be open minded in their expectations for his future.

Finally we should like to comment briefly on social relationships within the school. Although it is widely assumed that children do not like to be 'different', we have found that in the case of dyslexic children this assumption is highly questionable. Certainly we have met occasional children who did not like others at school to know about their difficulties. On the other hand, the obvious relief experienced by most children when told that they are dyslexic is sufficient evidence to suggest that dyslexia is seldom regarded by children as a stigma; and one teacher who works at a school which takes a proportion of dyslexic children has told us that, when he asked in a class, 'Who is dyslexic here?', the answer, 'Please sir, I am!' came from several of the class with positive pride! About seven boys from this school, aged between thirteen and sixteen, in fact volunteered recently to come and talk to a group of adults about their difficulties, and were able to do so with remarkable ease. On p. 13 we reproduce an attempt by one of these boys, aged sixteen, to explain in writing what he still finds difficult. His intention was simply to supply rough notes for his interviewer, but with his permission we are publishing what he wrote, both for its general interest and, in particular, as a demonstration of the way in which those with dyslexia can be fully articulate about their problems.

In general, it seems to us that if children wish to keep their dyslexia to themselves (as perhaps a small number do) that is up to them, provided they *themselves* understand their own limitations. Ideally, however, one looks for a climate of opinion where dyslexia is understood and accepted, and where there is no need for those who suffer from it to feel 'different' in any unpleasant sense. One teacher told us of a bright but severely dyslexic boy who was put into a class at school where the work was more academic: the first response of the other boys was, 'Why is *he* here?', but when the nature of his difficulties was explained they soon became sympathetic.

Moreover if a lecture on dyslexia is being given to adults there seems to us no reason at all why dyslexic children (if they are of an age to understand some of it) should not attend. The result may well be to give them a fuller appreciation of their problems, and nothing but good can come of this.

The main purpose of this chapter has been to call attention to the effect which dyslexia can have on the morale of a child and on that of his family and teachers. We do not wish to minimise the suffering which is sometimes involved, but there is no need for the child's life to be made a misery. Special teaching is required, and it is of course important that his difficulties should be understood. What is also important is that he

numbers I can do Them now bout
I am still qute bad.-

I could not prounce words like dislexer
bat now I can bat Some I never can Like
crosslaturel labatry.

I can not lean Things off by heart.

I ued to uniet The word prep "perp"
But now I do not So often.

I get bnudled up with ~~where~~
were and where.

I am no good at maths.

I am better at Reading but I ued to
miss a line or miss prounce Some
thing qute often

Sample 1 Notes made by Christopher B., aged sixteen.

13

should *know* that they are understood and that, whatever else happens, the dyslexia should not be allowed to damage his self-respect.

CHAPTER 3

The junior school age

It is perhaps a weakness of *On helping the dyslexic child* that it did not give sufficient consideration to the needs of the child of junior school age (8-11). Now that dyslexia is more widely recognised, however, there is a good chance that those who suffer from it will be picked out at an earlier age than hitherto, and it is, of course, an enormous advantage if the child is over the worst of his difficulties before he reaches the secondary school. In this chapter we shall draw on our recent experiences with these younger children.

Reading

The first priority with a dyslexic child of eight or nine is usually to improve his reading. Not only does weakness at reading affect all his school work and cripple his progress in almost all school subjects; it also limits his experience outside school. In countless ways he is not being stimulated. The result is that he is continually missing the opportunity to learn what is going on in the world around him. He fails to notice, for instance, the range of bus services in his home area, and he has no reason to wonder why mail vans have *'Royal'* written on them. Separately these points may seem trivial, but cumulatively the loss of experience is considerable.

For improvement in reading the most important thing is regular practice. He should, of course, be encouraged to read aloud so that you can correct his mistakes; and we recommend that the reading should take place at the start of the lesson when he is fresh, and that it should continue for as long as he can manage without fatigue.

It is also particularly important that he should have the right book. The right book for a particular child is one which deals with subjects in which he is already interested — Christmas, Guy Fawkes day, football, cars, aeroplanes, or whatever it may be. It is essential that it should be short — one that can be read in three or four sessions at most. If he is labouring so hard at reading that he cannot follow the story, good illustrations may help. The book should have really simple vocabulary, without the subject-matter being at too young a level. 'Babyish' material will bore him, while if the vocabulary is too hard he may guess wildly from the context, and this will encourage him in the habit of failing to look at words closely. Details of possible books are given on p. 17.

Not all the books which you choose in this way will be gems of literature. This need not cause you concern. More imaginative books, or the classics that you feel he should not be missing, can for the time being be *read to him*. Parents can do much here to enrich his experience and even to help him through a book that is on the long side. They can convince him that books are worthwhile and need not always be the occasion for tears and frustration.

When he is reading to you he may tire rather easily. Yet on the other hand he will probably take time to settle down. One has therefore to go on long enough for him to produce a concentrated effort, yet watch for the signs of fatigue which indicate that nothing more will be gained if he is pressed further.

It may be useful at this point to mention a few of the difficulties which he is likely to have in reading and to suggest ways of overcoming them. It is quite likely that his attention may slip to a line further down the page, in which case he will leave out what comes between. To rectify this he can be given a 'marker' (compare *On helping the dyslexic child*, p. 26). This is a piece of card like a short ruler. If it is placed under the line which he is reading, the lines below will not distract him. This placing is best done by the teacher at first, since the child himself has enough to think about. As he progresses it can be put somewhat lower — perhaps two lines ahead — so that he can see how soon the sentence ends, whether it is a question or not, and so on. Eventually he will no longer need it. If for a while after discarding it he occasionally uses his finger instead, one need not worry; at this stage it is unlikely to become a habit or slow down his reading unduly. In any case slow, accurate reading is preferable in remedial sessions to wild guessing.

He may also lose his place horizontally and read the letters of a word in the wrong order. This can occur even when the word is quite short. For many dyslexic children it is not easy to appreciate that the first letter of a word is the letter on the left! It may therefore be helpful if you ask, Which is the first letter? (In the case of certain combinations, e.g. *sh, ch,* and *th,* it is perhaps preferable to ask him what are the first *two* letters, since in certain circumstances two consonants should be thought of as a single unit. See p. 23.)

Sometimes he will fail to grasp the *structure* of a word and cannot start to read it simply because he cannot tell how much of it belongs to one 'mouthful', as it were, i.e. to a particular syllable. Here the marker can come in handy again. If a square piece is cut out of its top left corner, it can be so placed that only the first syllable, e.g. the *pro-* in *provide,* is showing; the rest of the word, being concealed, can be forgotten until the first syllable has been pronounced. He will gradually learn that *pro* is often a 'mouthful' on its own. Similarly the word *raced* can often be puzzling. If the *d* is covered, however, the word is immediately recognised as a word of the *a-e* type (see On helping the dyslexic child, p. 44), and the *d* can then be shown to be something tacked on the end.

At this stage he is very likely to misread or omit words. If he does, it may be helpful to use the marker to cover over other parts of the text which are not needed, or indeed simply to point to the words in question; in either case you are calling his attention to the fact that something has to be corrected. It is a common temptation for the teacher to rush in too hastily with the right answer and in our experience a little silent help of the kind described may enable the child to arrive at the right answer himself without being told. In addition he may sometimes rush in too hastily with the right answer, and in our experience a little you can take the pressure off him by assuring him that there is no need to hurry and that he can take his time!

You may also find that at this stage progress at reading outstrips progress at spelling. In particular there are certain short familiar words which he will manage to read but which he cannot be taught to spell because they are phonetically irregular, e.g. *great, laugh, early.* This need not cause you concern. In due course (it need not be soon) you will be able to discuss the spelling of these 'awkward' words with him. By then reading will have become easier and the experience which he has gained from learning to spell regular words can be used to help him to look carefully at the unexpected letters in irregular ones. He will notice what it is that is 'awkward' about them, and this will help him to remember them better. At a younger age, however, it is quite common for a dyslexic child to be able to recognise a word at sight without being able to spell it.

In the case of regular words it is useful if one can keep reminding him of the link between reading and spelling. Thus if he has recently been learning the spelling of *ai* words and he meets, say, the word *rain* in his reader, it is worth calling his attention to the *ai* in the spelling.

We end this section with some suggestions as to possible readers.

In our experience books from the following series are particularly likely to be enjoyed: the *Griffin Readers* and the *Dragon Books* by S.K. McCullagh (published by E.J. Arnold & Son), the *Oxford Colour Reading Books* (published by the Oxford University Press), the *Discovery Readers* by John Anderson (published by George Harrap & Co.), and *Bonfire Night* and *London Express* by J.E. Miles (Ginn & Co.). We also recommend the *Windrush* books by Frederick Grice (Oxford University Press); these have a more extensive vocabulary than the others and therefore should not be introduced too early.

Children who are confused about sounds and their spellings can perhaps best be helped if they begin with books whose approach is basically 'phonic' as opposed to 'look-and-say'. In other words, rather than ask them to *look* at a whole word and then *say* it, one should present them with words which can be taken apart into separate letters or small groups of letters; they can then build the word up from knowledge of what sound a particular letter makes. Thus it is a mistake, if a child is dyslexic, to present him at too early a stage in his reading with words such as *ask, want,* or *done;* although these words are common the vowels in them are not sounded in the way one might expect, which to a dyslexic child is very confusing. In this connection we recommend in particular the *Essential Read-Spell* series, by F.J. Schonell (Macmillan & Co.), the *Royal Road* series by J.C. Daniels and H. Diack (Chatto and Windus), and the six *Look-Out Gang* books by M.B. Chaplin (Robert Gibson & Sons). These are all planned to introduce new sounds gradually In view of the special problems of the dyslexic child we think it best to avoid any series which sets out to introduce the more common words without consideration of whether these words are phonetically regular, e.g. the *Ladybird Key Words Reading Scheme* by W. Murray (Willis and Hepworth). Books which involve 'look-and-say' will encourage a dyslexic child to rely on guesswork in reading and will not give him the phonic background which he needs for spelling.

Handwriting

Not all dyslexic children need help with handwriting. Among the eight and nine-year-olds who have come to us, however, quite a number have displayed poor co-ordination in general and find particular difficulty in handling a pen or pencil. This means that, quite apart from their uncertainties over spelling, putting letters of any kind down on paper is really hard work.

For many of them it may be helpful to do writing patterns such as those described below. This task gives them practice at the basic movements of writing while at the same time providing them with the opportunity to create something artistic. Our experience is that they enjoy such an activity and that the quick success which they achieve acts as an encouragement. Such encouragement is particularly important at a time when success in reading — let alone success in spelling — still seems a long way off.

Such training in forming letters and moving the hand across the page is helpful for reading as well as writing, since both activities require the establishment of correct habits of progress from left to right.

When we write we make a number of movements which can be distinguished as follows:

1 We draw the pen straight down the page so as to make uprights.
2 We make circular movements from the wrist so as to form rounded letters.
3 We make short zigzag lines, as in *v, w,* and *x.*
4 Combined with 1, 2 and 3, we are all the time making a continuous movement from the elbow which takes the pen along the page from left to right.

To make all these complicated movements at once is difficult, particularly for the many dyslexic children who lack a clear sense of direction, and it is therefore helpful if they are practised separately. Any awkward position, e.g. one where the elbow is stuck out sideways,

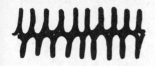

Fig. i

Fig. ia

Fig. ib

Fig. ii

Fig. iii

Fig. iv

Fig. v

Fig. vi

Sample 2 Writing patterns made by Christopher W., aged fifteen.

19

restricts the movements of the wrist and should be discouraged from the start.

On p. 19 Sample 2 shows some writing patterns which were specially made for this book by a dyslexic pupil.

The first pattern (Fig. i) combines simple uprights with continuous progress along the line. The *l* must be taken right up to the upper line and brought down vertically. (A *mild* slope may be permitted later in ordinary writing, but excessive slope crushes the rounded letters.)

To do these patterns a felt pen is very desirable, since it can be pushed in all directions quite easily. Also these pens are made in many delightful colours.

If the page is turned upside down when the child has completed the first row and a second row is now made touching the first one, a centipede-like design is obtained. This design, and all subsequent ones, can then be decorated in a variety of colours in whatever way the child pleases (Fig. ia). A different design can be obtained if the rows of *l*s are done the other way round so that the 'legs' meet; this is more difficult (Fig. ib).

The next pattern (Fig. ii) is a row of *o*s. This gives practice at forming rounded letters and joining them up. We have found that many children are careless in the way in which they link *o*s; if the join is made in the wrong place the *o* tends to look like an *a*. A row of *a*s in fact produces a slightly different pattern, and an interesting pattern can be formed by a row of *c*s, though it is not easy to make them regular.

More complicated patterns can be made if a row of the Fig. i pattern is alternated with a row of the Fig. ii pattern.

Fig. iii, a row of *d*s, is obtained by combining the movements of Fig. i with those of Fig. ii. The letter *d* is a particularly good one to practise, since one can impress on the child that he should do the round part first. This means that he can then distinguish it from a *b* where the correct place to start is at the top. If he is in the habit of starting at the top for *both* letters he may move the pen or pencil down — and then not know whether to move it to the left or to the right! This kind of indecision can be avoided if the two letters, *b* and *d*, are produced in quite different ways.

Fig. iv is a zigzag pattern, which will form the basis for writing *v*, *w*, and *x*, and Fig. v is a humpy pattern, which will be used for *m* and *n*.

If alternate letters of different types are used, e.g. if a spiky letter, such as *v*, is followed by a rounded one, such as *e*, to make *ve*, some even more varied patterns can be produced (see Fig. vi).

f,s, and *r* are difficult letters in themselves and hard to link with other letters; it is therefore wise to leave them to the last. *g* and *y* cannot easily be linked either, and it is perhaps best in their case not to insist on any link at all. Where two letters frequently go together, e.g. *t* and *h*, they can be practised as a pair.

Regular practice with these writing patterns over a month or two is likely to make writing less laborious. Even after this time it may still be helpful if the child continues for a while to write his word-lists and sentences with a felt pen; this will enable the new movements to become grooved.

Spelling

The younger child may not be at all confident about the sounds made by different consonants, and it is therefore best to check up on these in detail before asking him to attempt whole words. The words in Section I of the Appendix (pp. 58-59) are designed in the first place to give practice at recognising all the consonants. We suggest that these words are said aloud to the child and that he be asked to indicate the first letter of each word (or the last letter in the case of the words *box, mix,* and *six*). He can do this either by choosing the correct letter among a group of plastic or cardboard letters on the table or by pointing to the correct one among several written on paper or on the blackboard; alternatively he can be asked to write down the letter which he hears. It is unnecessary at present to ask him to *name* the letters; what is required is to teach him to associate a particular letter with a particular sound, and for this purpose naming is an extra complication. Also it is unnecessary at this stage to require him to distinguish between small and capital letters.

The words in list (a) of Section I of the Appendix have been grouped so as to allow for easy comparison between those consonants which are most likely to be confused with each other. Thus one needs to make sure that the child can distinguish clearly between the *f-, v-,* and *th* -sounds (*fan, van, than*), between the *k-* (or hard *c-*) and hard *g* -sounds (*cot, got*), between the *p-* and *b* -sounds (*pit, bit*), between the *t-* and *d* -sounds (*tip, dip*), and between the *m-* and *n* -sounds (*met, net*). A

21

useful way of achieving this is for the teacher to present the sounds or words in pairs and ask the child to say if they are the same or different. For example, one might successively present the following pairs: *met - net, met - met, net - net,* and *net - met,* the correct responses being 'different', 'same', 'same' and 'different'. By this means one can check that the child has heard the letters correctly, without the complication of asking him to write or point to anything. It is, of course, good for the child's morale that he should be getting things consistently right, and the teacher has the reassurance that the programme is being based on firm foundations.

The same technique can in fact be used at all stages, since it is applicable to any situation where two things need to be distinguished. The general procedure is that the child should be presented with a pair of words one of which — and not the other — exhibits a particular characteristic. Thus if at a later stage he has difficulty with triple consonants he can be asked if *spit* and *split* are 'the same' or 'different'; if he has difficulty with the 'grunting' *n*, e.g. if he spells *land* as *l-a-d*, he can be given the words *lad* and *land* and asked to say whether or not the *n* -sound is present. If he can learn to make distinctions in a simplified situation it will be easier for him to do so in more complex situations where there are other things to remember, whereas if he has too much to think about all at once he is likely to become confused.

It is possible that he will not be familiar with the less common consonants, viz. *j, v, w, x,* and *y,* in which case they will need to be explained to him. In connection with *x* one can point out that, although it has the same sound as *-cks,* it is used as an ending when there is one thing (e.g. *box*), whereas *-cks* is used when there are several (e.g. *clocks*). After teaching the consonant-sound of *y* at the beginning of a word, as in *yes,* it is important to mention that at the end of a word it has a short *i* -sound, as in *Betty,* since this is something which he will often meet in his reading.

The next step is to introduce the vowels, *a, e, i, o,* and *u.* It has to be stressed that these are special letters and are different from the others which he has been learning. There is no harm in using the word vowel if the child understands it, but one cannot count on its being familiar to all children of this age. The special nature of the vowels can be emphasised if one uses colour or produces bigger letters or letters made of a different material. One can explain that in the little words which he has been using the vowel is in the middle; like chocolates, these words have a centre, the consonants being like the chocolate on either side. One can add that in some very short words (e.g. *it, on, at*) there is no piece of 'chocolate' at the beginning and that in these cases we need to start with the vowel.

When he has understood this he will be ready to learn the individual sounds of the short vowels, ă, ĕ, ĭ, ŏ, and ŭ, and to sort words into lists as recommended in *On helping the dyslexic child,* p. 43. The words in the Appendix, (Section I, list (a), p. 58) can also be used for this purpose. Much of this work should be done orally or with the use of plastic or cardboard letters; even whole words can be written on cards by the teacher, so that the child has only to sort them into the correct column. At this age writing is likely to be laborious for him, and these other activities provide the necessary variety.

The next step is to teach those combinations of consonants which make only one sound (see Appendix, Section I, list (b), p. 59). The main ones are *sh, ch, th, qu, wh,* and *ck.* It is useful to have each of these combinations written on a single piece of card, so that when the child is building up words he can pick up the whole combination together. This helps him to think of it as one unit rather than as two separate letters. In the case of *wh* one should not perhaps insist on any difference of sound from *w*, since this is generally disregarded in speech; one can simply explain that there are a few words which begin with *wh* instead of *w*, especially words which ask questions. *When* and *which* are suitable for inclusion in the initial lists since they both have a short vowel; *whisk* is also suitable if the child knows the word. Other words beginning with *wh* will probably be remembered best if they are added to appropriate lists when the time comes, e.g. *whale* and *white* when the child is doing silent *e*, *wheel* and *wheat* when he is doing *ea* and *ee* words, and so on. The most common *wh* words are in fact the question- words, *when, which, why, what, where,* and *who,* along with *whisk, whale, white, wheat, whisper,* and *whistle.* The combination *ch* may also raise problems for the teacher; this is because at quite an early stage the child in his reading may meet words where *ch* is pronounced as *k*, e.g. *Christmas, Christopher, choir, chorus, chord, chemist, ache, echo,* and *anchor.* All such words, however, are too difficult to be included in spelling lists at this stage, and our suggestion is that you refer to the special pronunciation of *ch* only if it seems necessary to do so during the child's reading.

More help for dyslexic children

Practice is also needed in distinguishing two consonants where these have distinct sounds, such as *sp, dr* and *cl*. Examples are given in the Appendix, Section I, list (c), p. 59. Here it is necessary for the child to listen with particular care. This applies even more where there are three distinct sounds, such as *str* and *spl* (see Appendix, Section I, list (d), p. 60). If the short words in this section of the Appendix are practised at an early stage, the child will have less difficulty when he meets these combinations of letters in longer words, such as *instruction*.

Section I of the Appendix, list (e), p. 60, also gives practice at recognising combinations found at the end of words (*-ff, -ss, -lk,* etc), but these may be left until later if this seems more convenient.

The basic skill of learning to match sounds and symbols takes time; and it may be that quite a number of lessons will have passed before all the consonant sounds are known and can be written confidently. It may therefore be some time before one can start on words having a final *e* (See *On helping the dyslexic child* p. 44). Indeed the total programme outlined in *On helping the dyslexic child* may take up to two years with these younger children; if one rushes through the lists and exercises too quickly a large amount will be forgotten and there will be the frustration of continually having to 'go back'. Firm foundations and continuous revision are essential, and these are hard to achieve unless one goes very slowly.

At this age it seems undesirable to spend too much time doing sentences. At suitable intervals the child can be given specially devised ones (such as those in *On helping the dyslexic child*) as a check that a particular lesson has been learned; but he is likely to become bored if they are a regular feature of every lesson.

In *On helping the dyslexic child* the two ways of spelling the long *e* -sound, viz. *ee* and *ea,* are put on the same page (see p. 44). To the very young child, however, it may seem bewildering that the same sound can be spelled in more than one way, and it is perhaps preferable if *ee* and *ea* words are kept quite separate and presented on separate occasions. The fact that there is more than one way of spelling the long *e,* the long *a*, and the long *o* can be explained later when the child is in a better position to understand.

The irregular words given on p. 45 on *On helping the dyslexic child* (*who, where, could, have,* etc.) are likely to be difficult for the younger child even if he has learned the regular words thoroughly, and still more

24

so the irregular words on p. 51 (days of the week, etc.). It will probably be necessary to keep returning to them at suitable intervals, while the other material in *On helping the dyslexic child* is being consolidated.

Once the child has grasped the idea that the same sound can be spelled in different ways, it may be helpful to abandon what is called in *On helping the dyslexic child* his 'dictionary' of words and make a fresh start with a reporter's notebook in which the material can be arranged more concisely. On each page he can have two (or, at most, three) columns: the first page could be headed *a-e* and *ai* and would have lists of words of both types. Other pages could be headed *o-e* and *oa; ou* and *ow; er, ir* and *ur*, etc. In these columns he would first put, as a pattern, the words which he learnt in *On helping the dyslexic child* and then add other words of the same type as he himself meets them. As a result it will become a personal vocabulary book; the words in it will be words which he himself finds that he needs, and they will be sorted according to the principles which he has mastered. This will also serve to impress on him what these principles are, so that as new words turn up he will be able to add them to the page where they belong.

During this process he will come across words such as *sail* and *sale* which sound the same but which are spelled in different ways. Here he can have great fun decorating his notebook with illustrations showing the difference. Since it is his own personal notebook he is free to use his imagination. One pupil of ours, for example, drew on the left side of the page a fine *whale* spouting water, while on the right side, beside the word *wail*, there was simply the picture of a pram (with no occupant visible); and there were shrieks of mirth over this!

Further lists can be included from the present book, especially those given in Section II of the Appendix (pp. 60-61), viz. *-ue* and *-ew, -au* and *-aw, -ey* and *-ei*, etc. He can also make new lists which are a development of earlier ones. For example, after the page which contains *a-e* and *ai* words, he may like to make special lists of words ending in *-are* and *-air*, e.g. *spare* and *fair*, which involve the same combinations of letters but with an *r* added. Similarly, after the *o-e* / *-oa* page, there could be a page of words ending *-ore* and *-oar*, where again an *r* is added. Suitable words will be found in Section II of the Appendix, p. 62. At the end of the notebook he may like to include lists of words arranged according to the different endings discussed in Chapter 5.

While he is steadily working through this programme over a year or two, he can of course be encouraged to do free writing at school and can be given credit for imaginative ideas; indeed it may be helpful to have an explicit agreement between child and class-teacher that, when he does free writing, errors in spelling will not be penalised. In the special remedial lessons, of course, the position is quite different. The role of the spelling teacher (i.e. yourself) is to give the child words which he already knows how to tackle; and in this context it is essential to insist on full accuracy. It is important that these two types of situation should be kept quite distinct and that both child and teacher should know the difference between them. Indeed, even if in fact (as may happen) you yourself are the class teacher, who is at special times giving extra remedial lessons, both you and the child should be aware of the two different sets of requirements: in the one case the aim is imaginative writing, without too much distraction by worries over spelling; in the other case it is clearly understood that only manageable words will be given and that the child is expected to get them right.

In addition to his reporter's notebook for word lists he may also be given an index book in which words can be arranged alphabetically. In this he can put a few individual 'awkward' words which he meets in reading. It is most important, however, that this book should not become 'clogged up' with too many words. Only the common 'awkward' words should be included, or words which he is particularly likely to need; and he will find it helpful if the 'awkward' bit is picked out in some way, perhaps by suitable colouring or by ringing, as in *ne(ph)ew, w(or)d, br(ea)k.* Since they are likely to occur again and again he can continually look these words up and note what the difficulty is without being expected actually to learn them. For the present it is inadvisable to include in this index book 'awkward' words which are more than two syllables long.

This is perhaps the stage at which you can conveniently show him how to use a dictionary. It should, of course, be a simple children's dictionary, in which he will meet only words which are familiar to him and which are not too difficult to read.

It is important that he should not come to think of a dictionary simply as a device by means of which he can look up correct spellings. For such a purpose it would in fact be very inefficient, since at an early age he may not be in a position to set about finding the words which he needs, and if he develops the habit of looking up word after word he is in any case unlikely to remember more than a few of them. The main purpose in teaching children to use a dictionary is to give them a means of understanding the English language; for example, they may come as a result to think more fully about definitions, about synonyms, and about words derived from the same root. It is, of course, particularly desirable that they should have learned how to use a dictionary before they meet the technical terms which will be introduced to them at the secondary school stage.

To gain the most advantage from a dictionary the child needs to have acquired the basic knowledge of what letters can represent what sounds; then, if he is unsure how a particular word is spelled, he can try out a number of possible spellings from a restricted choice and have some chance of finding the word.

A further difficulty is that he may not know his alphabet. There seems no special merit in requiring him to recite the letters of the alphabet in order; this is the kind of sequencing task which dyslexic children sometimes find difficult, and even if they were eventually successful it does not follow that they would then know which way to turn the pages in order to find a particular letter, since this is quite a different task. It may help if a chart of the alphabet is put before the child with the letters arranged in groups of, say, five or six. If he learns the first five letters, A B C D E, and the last five, V W X Y Z, he will know whether to look at the beginning, middle, or end of his chart for the letter which he needs, and he can thus work out approximately where in the dictionary to look. When he has found his way to the first letter of the word he will need to repeat the procedure for the second letter and afterwards for the third. We suggest, therefore, that he memorises the first three letters of the word before he opens the dictionary at all; in most cases this will be sufficient to enable him to discover the word, and even those dyslexic children who are weak at tasks involving short-term memory will not find the task beyond them if no more than three letters have to be held in mind at once. If a fourth letter is needed he can return to the original word and work out its fourth letter, but he should be quite clear as to what are the first three letters before he does so.

Our experience is that dyslexic children can learn to derive benefit from a dictionary provided they are given tasks which are manageable for them, but it is important to remember that the skills involved are complex and should not be taken for granted.

Finally, here are three general rules, suitable for introduction to the child at this stage, which may help both his reading and his spelling.

i The first rule concerns *c* and *g*. These letters are normally *hard before a, o, and u and soft before e, i, and y*, e.g. *cat, cot, cut, game, go, gun, cent, city, cycle, gentle, gipsy* and *gym*. They are also hard before a consonant, as in *clip* and *green*. The difference between 'hard' and 'soft' can easily be shown to the child by means of examples, and the words 'hard' and 'soft' can then be introduced as the way of describing this difference.

At a suitable point you may like to call his attention to the few common words which are exceptions to this rule. The main ones are *give, gift, get, begin* and *girl*, along with a few words which end in -nger, such as *hunger, finger,* and *anger*.

It is possible to make a *g* hard before *e* or *i* by putting in the letter *u*, as in *guest* and *guilt*. Similarly, to make a *g* soft before *o* one can insert an *e*, as in *pigeon, dungeon,* and *George*. Again, if a hard *c*-sound is needed before *e* and *i* it is necessary to put a *k*, while if a soft *c*-sound is needed before *a, o,* or *u* one has to use an *s*. An alternative way of producing the soft *g* sound before *a, o* or *u* is to use a *j*. You can explain these points to the child as you come across them in reading.

ii The second rule concerns the doubling of consonants in two-syllable words. There are many words in English with double consonants in the middle, all of them having a strong emphasis on the first syllable and none on the second syllable, e.g. *bútter, bóttle*. The rule here is that *unless one doubles the middle consonant the first vowel will become long*.

Examples are given in Section III of the Appendix (p. 63), e.g. *kĭpper/wĭper, hŏpping/hōping, sǎddle/crādle*, and many others. Such words have a variety of different endings. A useful exercise is to take words from the two columns of p. 63 and ask the child to spell them. At first it may help him if you go alternatively from one column to the other; he then knows that he must pass alternatively from double consonant to single consonant. When he can do this with no difficulty you may like to choose words at random from the two columns; he then has to check for himself whether the vowel is short or long and put a single or double consonant accordingly.

iii The third rule enables him to tell whether to put *k* or *ck* and whether to put *ch* or *tch*. Here, too, the decision depends on whether the preceding vowel is short or long; where there is a short vowel then, once again, an extra consonant is needed.

Thus *back, neck, stick, lock* and *duck* all have short vowels, and the correct spelling is therefore *ck; make, like* and *poke* all have long vowels, and the correct spelling is therefore *k* with the silent *e* at the end. If there are two vowels together they count as a single long vowel; this means that in words such as *week, speak,* and *soak* a *k* is needed.

Similarly *match, stretch, pitch, Scotch,* and *Dutch* have short vowels, and the correct spelling is therefore *tch; beach, poach,* and *pouch* have two vowels, and the correct spelling is therefore 'ch'. The only important exceptions in this case are *much, such, rich, which, attach,* and the tiresomely irregular word *touch*.

All these rules can be taught not only during spelling sessions but in reading sessions also. In the course of reading the child will constantly have to consider whether to pronounce a *c* or *g* as hard or soft or whether a particular word is, say, *hopped* or *hoped*. He is likely to find it helpful in general if during reading sessions you call his attention to rules which you have already shown him as part of his training in spelling. Our experience is that teaching a child to spell helps his reading.

CHAPTER FOUR

A fresh start for the older child

Although there is a greater chance now than there was a few years ago that a child's dyslexia will be picked out at an early age, you may still meet children aged ten and more in whose case it has been missed. This can happen, for instance, when an extremely bright ten-year old has taught himself to read up to, say, the nine-year level. Everyone then assumes that his intellectual ability is mediocre; he is regarded as being neither weak enough for a special remedial class nor strong enough for an academic-type course. We have met several such children who were experiencing utter frustration in a C or D stream when they had enough ability to be in an A stream.

Once it is realised that they are dyslexic there is the opportunity for a fresh start.

Unfortunately this often means that a large number of existing habits will have to be changed. They may well have become discouraged from making an effort because their efforts in the past brought adverse criticism and not praise; they may have been put off reading exciting stories because of the very hard work involved, and in some cases they may have been so bewildered by failure that they have lost all self-confidence.

We are in no doubt that the correct procedure in these cases is to go back to the very beginning. They need to be shown consonants, pairs of consonants, and vowels in precisely the ways which we have described in Chapter Three. If this seems childish, the reason for it can be explained to them. One of the essential needs for a dyslexic child is that the teaching programme should be systematic and cumulative; without firm foundations there is no point in passing to more advanced work. It is probable, of course, that you will be able to move more quickly than you would in the case of an eight or nine-year old, but even with the older dyslexic child it is a mistake to take too much for granted.

By way of illustration here is some spelling from the exercise book of a boy aged thirteen.

The Fog

I wos worcing down the strete wen the fog cam down I Herd a screm But I cold not sea anething I Herd fot steps be hind me sum thing tucht my sholder I Did not turn I dust ran I cold not se were I wose gowing I cept Banging into peple. I cod Here my fotsteps ecow as I ran the water was drepieng from the arch it ecode I was scerd I turnd and cept runing I bumt into a tort ('tall'?) man with a Black bag and stic He sed wocth were yor gowing in an angery voys he hit me weth his stic hord on my back sow I grad his stic and thoo it away he shouted But I ran He ran after me He cort me and pold a long surfieel (?) nife from his dag (changed to 'bag') just as He was ad (crossed out) about to stab me I wock up, it was orl a drem. in the paper I sor the Hedlins. Jack the riper on the proul.

When this boy was given a traditional intelligence test the result was truly remarkable: in one of the items his score placed him in the top three of any thousand children of his own age-group.

How, then, would one start to teach him to spell? It is certainly not enough simply to correct the mistakes in this passage and hope that he will remember the correct spelling in the future. Nor is it enough (though it would be along the right lines) to correct 'worcing' to *walking* and give him *talking* and *stalking* at the same time. The truth is rather that he should never in the first place have been put into a position where these mistakes occurred; the ideal is to forestall mistakes rather than give corrective information afterwards.

If, however, for some reason, you were asked to comment on this piece of writing, our suggestion is that you should treat it as a piece of 'free composition' (compare p. 26). Since the boy has clearly put enormous effort into the story, you can express appreciation of this and congratulate him on producing something of such interest, without damping his enthusiasm by making adverse comments about the spelling. To teach spelling it is necessary to start somewhere quite different, viz. at a very much earlier stage.

The comments which follow are not offered, therefore, as suggestions for putting right the mistakes made by the boy in this particular context. Our intention is rather to invite the reader to consider the kinds of mistake which were made and to ask himself what background training is needed if such mistakes are to be avoided. It is important, as we said earlier (p. 8), that the teacher should be able to 'read the signs'; whatever the mistakes, he should be able to deduce from them what was lacking from the child's original training. In this case what is called for is a return to the basic elementary rules. These should be shown to the child one by one over a period of weeks, and only when he has mastered an easy rule should a more complicated one be introduced.

It may perhaps be helpful if we give particular examples. Thus at one point this boy spells *threw* as 'thoo'. This means that the teacher cannot take for granted that he knows the combinations of consonants given in Section I (c) and Section I (d) of the Appendix (pp. 59-60). It would be wise, therefore, not only to give him practice at words beginning *thr* but to check that he can spell easy words which start *br, cr, scr,* etc. That they should be easy is very important. Thus one might give him *scrub* or *scrap;* one would not give him *scratch* because there is the extra complication of whether to put *ch* or *tch* which cannot conveniently be mentioned until later (compare p. 29). Similarly one would not give him *threw*, since the *-ew* ending is again too complicated to introduce at this stage. Provided he knows the *-sh, -ft,* and *-st* endings one could give him the words *thrash, thrift,* and *thrust* and, after practice, intermingle them with *thud, thing,* and *thin;* only when he is getting them all right could one be sure that he is distinguishing those words which have the *r* after the *th* from those which do not.

The fact that he writes 'dust' for *just* shows that he needs practice at distinguishing *d* and *j*. The pairs *dot / jot* and *dab / jab* would be suitable here. Similarly the spelling 'wen' indicates that he needs practice at the combination *wh* (p. 23).

It is plain, too, that he is insecure over vowels. Even the ĭ- sound (short *i*) is misrepresented in the spelling 'drepieng' for *dripping;* and his mistakes over *street, scream,* and *see* ('strete', 'screm', 'sea' and 'se') show that he does not regularly represent the ē- sound (long *e*) correctly. The fact that he puts 'wock' for *woke* and 'lin' for *line* (in the attempt to spell *headline*) indicates the need to return to the initial vowel sounds which are given on pp. 43 and 44 of *On helping the dyslexic child.*

Later he can be shown the endings *-ing* and *-ed,* and he will then be in a position to spell *going* and *bumped* ('gowing' and 'bumt'). If he is told in addition that after a short vowel the consonant is doubled (p. 28), there will be no reason for any mistake over *dripping, grabbed* or *Ripper* ('drepeing', 'grad' and 'riper').

Once he knows the rule about when to put *ck* and when to put *k* (p. 29), this will cover him for the correct spelling of *stick* and *woke* ('stic and 'wock'). The rule that *c* is soft when followed by *e* would give him *kept* instead of 'cept', while the *-ce* ending discussed on pp. 39-40 would have enabled him to work out *voice* ('voys'). *Caught* ('cort') is given on p. 47 of *On helping the dyslexic child,* and the irregular *could* and *some* are given on the same page ('cold' and 'sum'). *All* ('orl') is given on p. 49 of *On helping the dyslexic child* while *scared* ('scerd') could be deduced from *scare* on p. 62. Even *echo* is mentioned in this book (p. 23) because of the hard *ch,* though one would probably decide that *echoed* ('ecode') is too rare and awkward a word to spend time on. Only a few words are left, therefore, which need to be specially noted as irregular; they are *said, people, watch, touched, pulled* and *heard.* In these cases it is, of course, the unusual representation of the vowel sound which causes the difficulty, and it is important for the teacher to make clear that failure to remember the spelling of these words is not reprehensible.

In general, we urge that older children whose dyslexia has only just been recognised should be taken back to the early stages and given a fresh start. It is unwise to attempt more advanced work until the foundations are fully secure.

We have one other suggestion for such children, viz. that they should practise their spelling on a typewriter. We have not used this method at all extensively, only on three boys in fact; the impression was that two of them were clearly helped, while the third was not a genuine failure since he was in a low state of morale at the time and various techniques had failed to arouse his enthusiasm. The advantages of a typewriter seem to be these. i Even for older dyslexic children handwriting may still be a problem, and if they are encouraged to type there is one less thing to worry about. Typing, unlike handwriting, does not involve detailed awareness of spatial relationships; the person does not have to remember at what angle to place the stroke or how far to continue with it, since the main requirement is simply to press the correct key. ii Because the typewriter operates on a 'one-letter-at-a-time' basis (at least unless one is very skilled!), the child has no alternative but to break the material up into single units; this seems a thoroughly good habit for those — including dyslexic children in particular — who have difficulty in dealing with larger units. iii The child can take his time. Indeed the use of the typewriter forces him to do so, since after pressing down a particular key he has to stop and consider carefully what key to press next. It will be possible for him to read the letters which he has typed so far; they are available and will not 'disappear' like auditory material, and by referring to them he can work out the exact point which he has reached. iv The result is often easier to read than handwriting. v There is the added advantage of novelty.

As a light-hearted game you may like to take over the typewriter yourself from time to time and to introduce some deliberate mistakes which the child is then asked to correct. This may help to train him to look at detail and to concentrate on accuracy rather than speed. On the few occasions when we have tried this procedure we found that it was enjoyed.

In spite of all that has been said, however, it is perhaps best to regard

the typewriter as a temporary makeshift which may contribute to
progress in the early stages. The ideal is that the child should learn to
produce legible handwriting and should be able to do so without too
much effort. This is a skill which it is quite possible for him to acquire
even at a later age, and when he can write fluently typing will no longer
be necessary.

CHAPTER FIVE

Word – endings and word – beginnings

Introduction

The purpose of this chapter is to outline a programme suitable for the
next stage after a child has completed the lists and exercises in *On
helping the dyslexic child*. We are assuming that he is familiar by this
time with all the most common vowel sounds and that he will be able to
spell large numbers of short words provided they are phonetically
regular.

The lists in *On helping the dyslexic child* also included a number of
standard word-endings (or 'suffixes'), viz. *-y, -ly, -ing, -ed, -er, -le* and
-tion (see *On helping the dyslexic child* pp. 46-50). If the child is to
tackle longer words an explicit study of these endings now seems
required, along with various others, such as *-el, -ous, -ary*, etc. A similar
study can also be made of word-beginnings (or 'prefixes'). One can then
show the child that longer words are composed of several parts and that
both endings and beginnings contain standard combinations of letters
which can be remembered as a group.

The first part of the chapter will be devoted to word-endings — simple
ones in the first place and afterwards harder ones — and the final part of
the chapter will be concerned with word-beginnings. As a rough guide
it is suggested that the simpler word-endings should be studied at the
primary school stage, while the harder ones and the word-beginnings

should be given to children of eleven and over. The exact pace at which the teacher goes, however, will depend on the individual needs of the child; and even in the case of older pupils it may be necessary, particularly if their dyslexia has only recently come to light, to check that they have a thorough knowledge of the material in the early part of the chapter before they proceed any further. To suppose, without consideration of his special circumstances, that a dyslexic child 'ought' to have reached a certain level by a certain age may cause the teacher to have wrong expectations.

It is important that at each stage of the chapter the main text should be studied in conjunction with the word-lists in Section IV of the Appendix (pp. 64-69), or, where appropriate, with *On helping the dyslexic child*, pp. 43-50. We have not attempted, however, in these word-lists to meet every possible need which the child may have; the Appendix would in that case have been both impossibly long and very tedious. Where some general rule was available, for example the rule that words ending in the *ŭry* -sound, if they are adjectives, are more likely to end -*ary* rather than -*ery,* a special list of such adjectives seemed unnecessary. Only where there may be genuine doubt, for example whether a word should end -*ent* or -*ant,* did we think it necessary to prepare lists of some of the more common words of each sort. These lists can of course be added to whenever the child comes across other similar words which he needs to spell.

Throughout the Appendix *silent* letters have been printed in italics (as in *k*now and dau*gh*ter). It seems desirable, whenever a silent letter occurs, that the pupil's attention should be called to it.

In Section V of the Appendix we have provided sentences for practice. It seemed to us that this would be helpful in the case of words ending in the *shŭn* -sound (*suspicion, mention,* etc.) and also in the case of words ending in -*ous,* since for both sets of words the rules are somewhat complicated. If a pupil has difficulty in remembering other endings the teacher may wish to invent further sentences so as to give him the necessary practice. We are hesitant, however, to recommend extensive use of sentences. They do not help the pupil to appreciate good English and they limit him to specially selected words. Such limitation was necessary in the early stages of his training because of the scarcity of words which he could then be expected to spell (hence the emphasis on sentences in *On helping the dyslexic child*); but at an older age dictations involving unselected words are perhaps more appropriate.

The material in this chapter may seem somewhat formidable, particularly the later sections; and we should like once again to emphasise the importance of going slowly and of not presenting it in too large 'doses'.

Simpler word-endings

-y and -ly *

The letter *y* is, of course, exceptional in that it can be used both as a vowel and as a consonant. When it is used as a vowel it is usually short, as in *gladly*, although there are a few words, e.g. *fly, cry, fry*, where it is long. In either case however, when the verb-form requires *s*, as in the third-person singular, or *d*, as in the past tense, the *y* changes to *ie*: thus we have *cry, cries, cried*, and *hurry, hurries, hurried*. The same happens with a noun when it becomes plural, e.g. *berry, berries*. This rule does not apply, however, in the case of words ending in *-ay, -ey*, and *-oy;* thus we have e.g. *stay, stays, stayed, annoy, annoys, annoyed*, and similarly the plural of *abbey* is *abbeys*.

There are some words which sound as if they have a *-y* ending but whose spelling is *-ey*. These need to be specially noted, and a list of the more common ones has been provided in the Appendix, Section IV, Group A (p. 64).

When *-ly* is added to adjectives which already end in *-y* or *-ay*, the first *y* changes to *i* (e.g. *happy, happily; gay, gaily*).

With many words which involve these endings the child has to apply the rule given on p. 28 in order to decide whether to double the middle consonant or not, as in the following examples: *lāzy, hăppy, bŏnny, bòny, chăry, Hărry*.

-ing †

Where a word ends in *-ing* the previous vowel will again be long unless the consonant is doubled; for example, the *o* in *hoping* is long, while the *o* in *hopping* is short. When *-ing* is added to a word which ends in silent *e*, the silent *e* is no longer needed, since the *-ing* itself makes the original vowel long; thus despite the long *o, hoping* does not require an *e*.

---

* For lists see *On helping the dyslexic child*, pp. 46-47.
† For lists see *On helping the dyslexic child*, p. 47.

-ed ‡

We have sometimes found that when writing a past tense a child leaves out the *e*; thus *stayed* might be written as 'stayd' and *hoped* as 'hopd' (or even as 'hopt', since the sound of the word suggests a *t* at the end). Once he understands what a past tense is, however, it can then be explained that, with a few exceptions, past tenses end in *-ed*. (The exceptions are words such as *ran, saw,* and *caught* which are quite unlike the regular past tenses in sound). Thus, even though one cannot hear the *e* in words such as *stayed* and *hoped,* the *ed*-ending is needed, never *d* on its own.

The few cases where this rule does not apply require to be specially noted. The important ones are: *slept, crept, wept, paid,* and *made.* From the sound one might infer that the ending was *-ed*, as in the regular past tenses, but in fact it is not.

The addition of *-ed* has the same effect on the previous vowel as the addition of *-ing*, that of making it long. It is therefore necessary, once again, to apply the rule given on p. 28 to decide whether the consonant should be single (as in *hoped*) or double (as in *hopped*).

-er *

Like *-ing* and *-ed, -er* can also make the earlier vowel long; and doubling the consonant is again necessary if the vowel is to be kept short; thus *latter* has double *t*, *later* a single one.

-le and -el †

-le is a very common ending for short words. Many of them are nouns, e.g. *table, bottle;* some are verbs, e.g. *nibble, hobble,* and a very few are adjectives, in particular *little, middle,* and *double.* The pronunciation is approximately 'ŭl', and if the child is told that 'ŭl' -words normally end in *-le* he is unlikely to have any difficulty over the words on the list given in the Appendix, Section IV, Group B (p. 64). He may, however, need to be told that the rule about doubling the consonant after a short vowel applies in the case of these two-syllable words also, as, for instance, in *tāble* and *dăbble.*

There are some words, however, which end in *-el.* Since they are

---

‡ For lists see *On helping the dyslexic child,* p. 47.
* For lists, see *On helping the dyslexic child,* p. 49.
† For lists, see *On helping the dyslexic child,* p. 49.

much less common, it seems advisable not to start on them until the *-le* words have been mastered. When the time comes, however, one can explain to the child that some *'ŭl'* -words have *-el*, not *-le*. It is then possible to give him guidance as to which words go which way.

This can be done as follows: words which have a 'hard' consonant or an *f* before the ending have *-le*, whereas words with a 'soft' consonant before the ending have *-el*. The 'hard' consonants are *b, p, d, t, k,* hard *c,* and hard *g;* and 'soft' consonants are *ss, v, w, m, n,* soft *c,* and soft *g.* The child will already have met the difference between 'hard' and 'soft' *c* and *g* (p. 28), and he can now be shown that, in general, *ss, v, w, m,* and *n* make softer sounds than *b, p, d,* and *t.* After a hard consonant and an *f* the letter *l* (pronounced *'ŭl'*) is much easier to say than after soft consonants, and it can follow the consonant immediately with no difficulty in pronunciation; when the *'ŭl'* -sound follows a 'soft' consonant, however, pronunciation is difficult unless a vowel sound comes in between. This is why the *e* comes first when the consonant is soft. If the child is asked to say *table* and *towel* successively the difference will probably become clear to him. With soft *c* and soft *g* (as in *parcel* and *angel*) there must in any case be an *e* immediately afterwards so as to ensure that the *c* and *g* remain soft. The words on p. 64 have therefore been arranged to show the division between hard consonants and *f* (with *-le*) on the one hand and soft consonants (with *-el*) on the other. Below these two main lists we have given a list of exceptions of which there are only very few.

The *s-* and *z-* sounds may cause some doubt. Double-*z* counts as a hard letter, as in *dazzle,* while double-*s* is clearly soft, as in *tassel* and *vessel.* Where the *s* is followed by a silent *c* or *t* (as in *muscle* and *castle*) the spelling is *-le,* in deference, as it were, to the hard letters which are present but not pronounced. Where there is a single *z* or an *s* pronounced as a *z,* however, the spelling, surprisingly, is *-el,* as in *hazel* and *easel.* (The only common exception to this is *measles*). We are not, of course, talking here about words where the emphasis is on the *-el* ending, such as *hotél* and *expél;* no rules are needed for words of this kind, since the spelling must clearly be *-el* because of the sound.

A very common *-le* ending is *-able,* as in *probable;* also quite a number of words end in *-ible,* e.g. *possible.* In these cases we cannot hear the vowel distinctly because the emphasis is on the beginning of the word; we must therefore not go by what we hear but must simply bear in mind that the *'üble'* -sound is much more often spelled *-able* than *-ible*. It is the *-ible* words, therefore, which have to be remembered specially, and a list of the most common is to be found in the Appendix, Section IV, Group B (p. 65).

-tion ‡

Later experience has suggested to us that the *-tion* words given on p. 50 of *On helping the dyslexic child* were not altogether well chosen. Too many of them have turned out to be unfamiliar even to the older pupil, and they were not systematically organised in respect of length. The second printing of *On helping the dyslexic child* gives a revised list in which we have attempted to include only those words likely to be encountered by children of primary school age. When the *-tion* ending is taught to children of eleven and under it is important that the examples given should be words with which they are familiar. Later they can be shown the spelling of words ending in *-cion, -shion, -sion,* and *-ssion* (see pp. 42-43), but this should not be done just yet.

The s- or z- sound at the end of a word

To introduce these sounds you may find it helpful to call the child's attention to the fact that, although regular plurals simply involve the addition of *s*, this *s* is sometimes pronounced as though it were a *z*; thus although the plural of *clock, clocks,* has an *s*- sound, the plural of *hen, hens,* has a *z*- sound. Similarly the third-person singular of verbs is always spelled with *s* but is sometimes pronounced as though the *s* were a *z*, as in *begs*.

On other occasions when an *s*- or *z*- sound is heard, it is rarely spelled just *s* or just *z*. The child will need to consider first of all whether it is in fact an *s* -sound or a *z*- sound. When he has done this the following rules usually apply:

    i   If the *s* -sound follows a short vowel the spelling is usually *-ss* (double *s*), as in *less, kiss,* and *toss*. (The only common words having the *s*- sound and yet ending in single *s* are *gas, atlas, Christmas, this, thus, bus, plus,* and *minus*).

    ii   If the *s*- sound follows a long vowel or pair of vowels, the spelling at the end of the word will be either *-ce*, as in *face* and *peace*, or *-se* as in *case* and *house*.

‡   For lists, see *On helping the dyslexic child*, p. 50.

More help for dyslexic children

iii If the *z*- sound follows a short vowel, then the *z* is doubled, as in *fizz*.

iv If the *z*- sound follows a long vowel or pair of vowels, the spelling at the end of the word will be either *-ze*, as in *prize* and *freeze*, or *-se* as in *rise* and *choose*.

In brief, apart from plurals and the third-person singular of verbs, if there is an *s*- sound at the end of the word one writes either *-se* or *-ce;* if there is a *z*- sound one writes either *-se* or *-ze*. No attempt has been made to list all the words which exemplify this principle, since this would have made the Appendix too unwieldy.

It is also worth remembering that there are many longer words having the *s*-sound which end in *-ence* and *-ance,* such as *convenience* and *importance.* These are discussed on p. 47.

-ture

This ending is pronounced approximately *'cher'*, and the pupil can be told that to represent the *cher* -sound the spelling *ture* has the best chance of being right.

There are, however, a few words which end in the *'cher'* -sound but, instead of having the ending *ture,* are spelled exactly as they sound. Among the commonest are: *teacher, preacher, butcher, archer, stretcher,* and *voucher.* Any others will be found to derive from a verb ending in *ch*, with the additional *er* representing the person who does the activity in question, e.g. *poach, poacher.*

Lists of words in *-ture* are given in the Appendix, Section IV, Group C (p. 65).

Harder word-endings

The material presented so far in this chapter will normally be suitable for children under eleven. At secondary school, however, they are likely to meet new subjects which may have a technical vocabulary and are almost certain to make fresh demands in spelling. As a result they will meet longer words and will need to study more advanced endings.

We shall begin by considering the problems involved in the reading and spelling of longer words in general. Next we shall consider longer words with the *'shŭn'* -ending, after which the following new endings will be studied: *-age, -ace,* and *-ate; -ous; -al; -ary* and *-ery; -ent* and *-ant,* and *-ence* and *-ance.*

Longer words

We have continually found with dyslexic children that the actual
amount of material which they can handle at a given moment of time is
limited. When confronted with longer words they tend to 'lose the place'
and forget what point they have reached. Here are some typical mis-
spellings: 'temption' for *temptation,* 'alpcation' for *application,* and
'imagention' for *imagination.* Similarly a dyslexic child may be able to
say 'pre', 'lim', 'in', and 'ary' after the teacher provided he is able to
treat them as separate units; he may even be able to say 'prelimin. . . .'
followed by '. . . . .ary'. But if he tries to say *preliminary* (all at one
'go') he becomes confused. It is as though he cannot 'hold in mind' all
the separate parts of the word at once, and thus cannot be sure of getting
the parts in the right order.

Since one cannot assume that he will grow out of this limitation, it
follows that he will be helped in his spelling of longer words if a
standard and recognisable part of the word can be written as one unit.
This part of the problem can then, as it were, be put on one side while
he concentrates his attention on what comes next.

In the case of longer words the pupil should be encouraged to say
them aloud before attempting to spell them and to *count the number
of syllables.* This is a possible check against the omission or transposition
of letters; he can be encouraged to stop when he has completed a
syllable in writing and take stock of how many more syllables are needed. When a word is written down it can be inspected visually, and the
great advantage of visual material is that it 'stays put' and can be re-
examined later; auditory material, in contrast, has to be remembered
in its entirety or it will 'disappear'. The dyslexic child can use this fact
to his advantage by writing down the first syllable of a long word and
then concentrating his full attention on the next one; this saves him
having to overload himself by thinking of every syllable at once. If
necessary the 'unwanted' parts of the word can be covered over with the
hand or with a strip of cardboard.

Although omission of syllables is the more common type of error,
we have also occasionally come across spellings by dyslexic children
where the same syllable was put in twice, e.g. 'animimals' for *animals*
and 'conconset' for *concert.* This, too, seems to be an example of 'losing
one's place'; and counting the number of syllables seems again to be

the best safeguard against it.

As a general principle in teaching a dyslexic pupil to spell, we should like to suggest that prevention is better than cure. If he can be encouraged to work out in advance what is needed and apply the rules and procedures which he has been taught, this is far more satisfactory than that the teacher should wait for him to make mistakes and then correct them. In the case of longer words, however, it is sometimes possible, when he makes mistakes, to take the opportunity of showing him something about the effect of his dyslexia. This can be done as follows. Let us suppose, for example, that he spells *application* as 'alpcation'. In that case one can say to him, 'Tell me what you've put'. In all probability he will say 'application', perhaps wondering, from the tone of your voice, if he has made a mistake, but not examining what he has written closely. If, however, he is made to cover over all the word except the first three letters, *a-l-p,* he can easily read them as *'alp'*; similarly when he has covered the rest of the word over he can read the *'-ation'* at the end, and, when he is ready, can add the *c* -sound to it. This procedure enables him to know that he has in fact put 'alp-cation', and this is something which he could not possibly know by trying to study the word as a whole. One can then say to him, 'What is the target-word?' or 'What word were you *trying* to spell?', and then give him the chance to work out the necessary correction. Some pupils may be helped if one points out how this difficulty in monitoring what they have written is a special characteristic of dyslexia and that those who are not dyslexic can recognise 'at a glance' things which a dyslexic person can appreciate only by careful checking of each syllable. It may well be reassuring to some pupils if they are given this kind of indication of where their weakness lies.

The '**shun**' -ending

Once a pupil is familiar with the combination *-tion* he should be encouraged, when he needs to spell longer words, to listen for the sound *immediately before* the ending. In many cases this is a vowel, as in *indignation, commotion,* etc., and he is unlikely to have any problem in determing which vowel it is.

If it is a consonant, however, this may be more difficult, since consonants tend to combine with the *-sh* -sound in ways which may be unfamiliar to him. The important combinations seem to be *-ption* (as in *adoption*), -*ction* (as in *fiction*), -*stion* (as in *question*), -*ntion* (as in *mention*), and — most difficult of all — -*nction* (as in *junction*). Considerable practice may be needed before the pupil can pick out these combinations and letters every time. When he is able to do so, he will be able to give more concentration to the earlier syllables. This is one of the situations where he should be asked to count the number of syllables so as to make sure none are added or omitted.

There is a further complication which awaits the pupil when he has reached a more advanced stage: the same *'shun'* -sound can be spelled in other ways, viz. -*cion*, -*shion*, -*sion*, and -*ssion*. Lists of words with these different endings are given in the Appendix, Section IV, Group D (pp. 65-66).

-cion.

Fortunately there are only two words in -*cion*, viz. *suspicion* and *coercion;* and these can therefore be learned separately.

-shion.

Similarly there are only two words in -*shion*, viz. *cushion* and *fashion;* these also can be learned separately.

-sion.

With regard to -*sion*, the following guide-lines apply: **i** After *l* one finds only -*sion*, as in *compulsion*. **ii** After *n* or *r* one finds both -*sion* and -*tion*, as in *tension, version, attention, exertion*, etc., and a list of the most common words of each kind has therefore been provided on p. 65. **iii** Where there is the *'zhun'* -sound after a vowel, the correct spelling is always *'-sion',* as in *occasion* and *cohesion*.

-ssion.

The common -*ssion* words have been listed on p. 66.

Sentences have been provided on pp. 69-70 so as to give the pupil practice at recognising these somewhat complex differences.

-age, -ace, -ate

These three endings illustrate the fact that the last syllable in some English words is not fully pronounced, as in *damage, menace*, and *fortunate*. The sounds are approximately *'ŭj'* or *'ĭj'*, *'ŭs'*, and *'ŭt'*, but from these on their own it is not clear what vowel is needed.

The following guide-lines may be helpful: (**i**) nouns whose ending sounds like *'ŭj'* or *'ĭj'* often end in -*age;* (**ii**) nouns whose ending sounds like *'ŭs'* often end in -*ace;* (**iii**) adjectives whose ending sounds like *'ŭt'* often end in *-ate*. Lists of words are given in the Appendix, Section IV, Group E (p. 66).

Verbs ending in *-ate* are easier to deal with, since the long *a* is clearly sounded, as in *excavate.*

-ous

The ending *-ous* has much the same sound as the ending *-ace*. While most *-ace* words are nouns, however, most *-ous* words are adjectives.

In the Appendix (Section IV, Group F, p. 67) these adjectives have been classified into various groups. Words with a consonant before the *-ous* are the most straightforward, e.g. *famous,* and we have included in this list two words in *-geous* (*gorgeous* and *courageous*) where the function of the *e* before the *-ous* is simply to soften the *g*. Where there is an '*i* ' -sound (short *i*), before the *-ous, -ious* is likely to be right more often than *-eous,* but words with both kinds of ending have been listed for reference.

In the case of adjectives ending in *-tious* and *-cious* it may be helpful to draw a comparison with words which end *-tion* and *-cion.* Here the *ti* and *ci* are both ways of spelling the *sh* -sound; and in the same way, if an adjective ending in *-ous* has this *sh* -sound, the spelling is likely to be either *-tious* or *-cious. -cious* is in fact much more common than *-cion,* and of the adjectives which end in *-tious* (as opposed to *-cious*) the great majority are connected with a *-tion* noun; *ambitious,* for example, is connected with *ambition.*

If there is an *n* -sound before the *-shus* the word will always end *-tious,* as in *pretentious* or *licentious.*

If a *k* -sound occurs immediately before the *sh* -sound this *k* -sound may combine with the *s* -sound to form an *x* and we will get *xi*. The child who understands this point can therefore be warned to expect some words to end in *-xious,* the two main ones being *anxious* and *noxious.* He should remember, however, that *infectious* keeps the *cti,* as does the related noun, *infection.*

Sentences for practice are given in the Appendix, Section V (pp. 69-70).

-al

It is useful to leave an appreciable gap between doing the *-le/-el* endings (pp. 37-38 above) and doing words in *-al,* so as to avoid possible confusion between the two.

Most *-le* and *-el* words are nouns; in contrast words ending in *-al* are mainly adjectives. Thus if a word with the '*ŭl*' -sound at the end is an adjective there is a good chance that the spelling -*al* will be correct, as in *usual* or *original.* This general rule covers so many adjectives that it seemed to us unnecessary to list them separately in the Appendix. The only major group of exceptions are the words having a *b* before the '*ŭl*' -sound, where the ending is, of course, -*le,* e.g. *portable, possible.*

In the case of nouns having the '*ŭl*' -sound, however, the position is more complicated. Where the spelling is -*al,* these nouns can conveniently be divided into three classes:

i There are some nouns which are derived from verbs, e.g. *trial, denial, rehearsal, betrayal.* These are instantly recognisable from the fact that, when the '*ŭl*' -sound is removed, a familiar verb is left, e.g. *try, deny, rehearse, betray.* These words can helpfully be included in the pupil's notebook.

ii Quite a number of nouns in -*al* are also used as adjectives. In some cases both noun and adjective are likely to be familiar to the pupil, e.g. *general, corporal, material, moral.* There are other words, however, where the adjectival usage is not easily recognisable; thus the word *animal* is an adjective in the expression 'our animal nature' and the word *signal* is an adjective in the expression 'a signal success'. One must assume that only the very bright pupils will recognise the adjectival usage in these less obvious cases. In spite of this, however, it seemed to us helpful to collect together in the Appendix all the -*al* nouns which could ever function as adjectives (see Appendix, Section IV, Group G, p. 68); then if the pupil *knows* that they are also adjectives he will not need to learn them separately. Words in the list can then be distinguished from -*al* nouns which *never* function as adjectives, e.g. *sandal, rascal,* where the -*al* ending simply has to be learned. There seems no reason, for example, why *sandal* should be spelled -*al* and *candle* -*le.* Nouns in -*al* are, of course, far less numerous than nouns in -*le.*

A word which may cause special trouble is the word *principal.* Not only can it be both a noun (e.g. the Principal of a College) and an adjective (meaning 'chief'); it is also liable to be confused with the -*le* noun, *principle,* which means approximately 'rule'.

There is a possible difficulty over adjectives having the '*shŭl*'-sound at the end, e.g. *initial* and *crucial,* since from this sound on its own there is no means of knowing whether the spelling should be -*tial* or -*cial.* If the pupil is in doubt he has a better chance of success if he puts

-tial, since *-tial* words are the more common. Also, if there is an *n* before the *'shŭl'* -sound, the spelling will almost certainly be *-tial*, as in *essential, influential,* and *torrential.* (A helpful comparison can be made here with the *'shŭs'* -sound: when there is an *n* before this sound, the spelling is almost certain to be *-tious,* not *-cious,* as in *pretentious.* See p. 44.) We have found two exceptions to this rule, viz. *financial* and *provincial*; despite the *n* before the *'shŭl'* -sound both these words end in *-cial,* and they have therefore been listed in the Appendix (see Section IV, Group G, p. 68).

-ery and -ary, -ent and -ant, and -ence and -ance

In saying words of this kind one makes the somewhat 'nondescript' sounds *'ŭry', 'ŭnt',* and *'ŭnce'* with no clearly recognisable vowel. The following suggestions, however, may help the pupil to decide whether this 'nondescript' sound should be represented by *e* or *a.*

Words in **-ery**

   i   Many words in *-ery* express a sort of stock-in-trade of a trader, and the pupil will already know that the word for a person who 'does something' (such as trading) is likely to end in *-er.* Thus we have:

   grocer − grocery
   stationer − stationery (notepaper, etc.)
   cutler − cutlery
   collier − colliery
   robber − robbery

Also, even when there is not a word ending in *-er* for the 'agent', there may still be a reference to stock-in-trade or 'doing something' which justifies the use of *-ery.* Thus we have *embroidery, trickery, foolery, finery, mockery, cookery, bribery,* and *machinery.*

   ii   Where a word refers to a place of some kind *-ery* is the more likely ending, as in *gallery, shrubbery, rockery, Chancery, Deanery, nursery,* and *cemetery.*

   iii   There are adjectives in *-ery* which are connected with nouns in *-er.* Some of the more common ones are: *powdery, papery, feathery, coppery, silvery, thundery, watery,* and *peppery.* These adjectives mean 'like powder', 'like paper', etc. You may also like to call the pupil's attention to *fiery.*

Words in **-ary**

Where there is an adjective the ending *-ary* is far more likely than the ending *-ery*, as in *imaginary*, *necessary*, and *stationary* (in the sense of 'not moving').

There are also a few nouns which end in *-ary*, in particular *dictionary*, *boundary*, *constabulary*, and *dromedary*.

In some cases the pupil may be able to discover the correct vowel in an *ŭry* word by trying to find a connected word in which the vowel sound is clear. Thus *imaginary* is connected with *imagination*, where the *ā*-sound (long *a*) stands out; similarly *history* must be *-ory* because the word *historian* clearly carries an *o* (compare also *category*, *memory*, and *allegory*). By the same argument *stationery* (in the sense of 'notepaper'.) must end *-ery*, since *stationer* ends in *-er*.

All the above words can helpfully be included in the pupil's notebook.

Words in **-ent** and **-ant**
The rule about hard and soft *g* and *c* (p. 28) is of help in some cases: thus where there is hard *g* or hard *c* one can expect the ending *-ant*, as in *elegant*, *extravagant*, *significant*, and *applicant*, and where there is a soft *g* or soft *c* one can expect *-ent* (with the *e* keeping the *g* or *c* soft), as in *indulgent*, *intelligent*, *recent*, and *innocent*. (Very occasionally you may meet a word with a soft *g* which nevertheless ends in *-ant*, e.g. *pageant* and *sergeant*, and in these cases, of course, an *e* is needed after the *g* to keep it soft. Unless the child is very sophisticated, however, this is an extra complication which you will probably wish to ignore). The *s-* and *sh* -sounds go the same way as the soft *c* -sound and therefore require *-ent*, as in *effervescent*, *patient*, and *efficient*. *-ment* is a particularly common ending for nouns derived from verbs, e.g. *excitement* and *amusement*.

Words in **-ence** and **-ance**
The same principles apply in the case of words ending in *-ence* and *-ance*. As examples of words which obey the rule about hard and soft *g* or *c* may be cited *elegance*, *significance*, *intelligence*, and *adolescence*. Similarly where there is an *s-* or *sh* -sound the spelling is likely to be *-ence*, as in *essence* and *conscience*.

In the case of other words in this group there seems no alternative other than gradually learning them from the lists. Some of the more common nouns and adjectives in *-ent* and *-ant* are therefore set out in the Appendix (see Section IV, Group H, p. 69).

Word-beginnings

It may be of help to an intelligent dyslexic child to study not only
word-endings (or 'suffixes') but also word-beginnings (or 'prefixes'). The
lists which follow contain some of the more common prefixes. They
include both those prefixes which stay the same whatever letter comes
afterwards and some more difficult ones where the final consonant of
the prefix may be affected by the next letter in the word; thus the prefix *circum-* never changes, while the prefix *con-,* although it stays the
same before *f,* as in *confirm,* nevertheless changes to *m* before a *p* or *b,*
as in *compare* and *combine.* Our suggestion is that the pupil should
learn these prefixes in such a way that he can recognise them at once
when he reads them; he can then set off confidently, because of their
familiarity, when he has to spell a word which begins with one of them.

We have not included the basic meaning of these prefixes in the
present chapter nor any derivations, whether from Latin, Greek, or
Anglo-Saxon. To do so would have been to create an extra complication.
When a prefix occurs in a compound word, its meaning as part of the
compound may not be at all near its original meaning; for example, the
word *announce* involves the prefix *ad-,* but a knowledge that 'ad' in
Latin means 'towards' does not help a dyslexic child to spell the word
correctly. What is needed is *recognition* of prefixes for spelling purposes,
and this can be taught without troubling the pupil about their meanings.
If, however, the teacher wishes to make a more systematic study of
prefixes in general and what they mean, a comprehensive list will be
found in *Chambers 20th-Century Dictionary.*
We are assuming that the pupil is aged thirteen or more by the time
he has reached this point and that he is capable of reasonably advanced
work, e.g. CSE or O level English.

The prefixes *circum-, inter-, mis-,* and *per-* never change.
Some of the more common words having these prefixes are:

circumstances	interval	mistake	perfect
circumference	interlude	misfire	permit
circumscribe	interview	misunderstand	perfume
circumspect	interpreter	misplace	perform
circumvent	interloper	misbehave	percussion

It should be noted that the prefix *mis-* has only one *s*, unlike the short words of similar sound, e.g. *miss, kiss,* and *bliss.*

The prefixes *pre-, de-, re-,* and *pro-* also never change. Some of the more common words having these prefixes are:

prefect	decide	report	progress
prepare	depart	remark	pronoun
prefix	deceive	reward	product
preposition	detail	return	profess
prefer	determine	restrain	profit

These prefixes are awkward in that the sound of the word as spoken does not always indicate clearly what is the right vowel to use. Sometimes the sound is ē (long *e*) or ō (long *o*), as in *prefix* and *pronoun;* sometimes it is ĕ (short *e*) or ŏ (short *o*), as in *preposition* and *profit.* It seems best, therefore, that the pupil should learn what is the spelling of these prefixes rather than try to infer it from the sound.

The prefixes *en-, in-* and *con-* can be grouped together because they all end in *n*. Usually the *n* stays, but before *b* or *p* it changes to *m*. Examples are as follows:

Stays the same	*Changes*
engage	embrace
	emperor
inactive	imbibe
	impatient
confident	combine
	company

In the case of *in-* and *con-* before *l* and *r*, there is a doubling of the consonant, as in *illegal, irrigation, collect* and *correct.*

The prefixes *dis-* and *ex-* can be grouped together because of the *s* -sound at the end. Both of them stay the same before most letters, but when the next part of the word begins with an *f* the correct spelling is *ff* (double *-f*). Examples are as follows:

Stays the same	*Changes*
disappoint	difficult
dislike	different
exit	effort
expel	effect

More help for dyslexic children

The prefix *dys-* is rare. Its general sense is 'difficulty with . . .'; thus a person with *dyspepsia* has difficulty with digestion. This prefix would barely be worth mentioning were it not for the fact that the pupil may sometimes need to know how to spell *dyslexia!*

The prefix *sub-* remains the same except when it is followed by *c, g, f,* and *p.* In these cases the consonant doubles. Examples are as follows:

Stays the same	*Changes*
suburb	succeed, success
subway	suggest, suggestion
subsidence	suffer
	sufficient
	suppose
	support
	supply

There is no change when *sub-* is followed by the letter *m,* as in *submarine.* Although there are some words which start *summ-* (e.g. *summary, summit*), this double *m* is not caused by the prefix *sub-,* which is not present in these words.

Finally, the prefix *ad-* stays the same in a few cases, but more often gives rise to a doubling of the consonant. Examples are as follows:

Stays the same	*Changes*
adapt	abbreviate
adept	accord, accept, access, accent
adopt	affect, afflict, affair, affirm
—	aggressive, aggregate
adhere	allow, allotment, allocate
adjective	announce, annoy
admit	arrest, arrive, arrange
advice	assert, assist
	attend, attach, attempt, attack

Ad- before a *q* becomes *acq-,* as in *acquaint, acquiesce, acquire,* and *acquit.*

In general, *ad-* remains the same before vowels, *h, j, m,* and *v,* and leads to a doubling of the consonant before *b, c, f, g, l, n, r, s,* and *t.*

Where there is *no* doubling of the consonant before these letters (as in *abroad, aloft, ablaze, abreast*), this is because the word has nothing to do with the prefix *ad-* and there is therefore no *d* to be affected. It will be noticed that these four words (unlike the ones given above) would still be complete words even if the *a* at the start were taken away. This kind of *a* is in fact a different prefix and is not very common.

To call the pupil's attention to word-endings and word-beginnings is one way of encouraging him to look at words *in detail*. If he cannot absorb the whole word at once it is clearly better that he should break it down into manageable parts rather than make a wild guess.

CHAPTER SIX

Arithmetic

If a child has some of the problems of reading, spelling, sequencing and orientation characteristic of dyslexia, it is possible that he will also have difficulty with arithmetic. Indeed in some cases special coaching at arithmetic seems quite as necessary as special coaching at reading and spelling.

The position seems to vary, however, between one child and another. In our experience quite a number of dyslexic children make mistakes over arithmetic simply because they lack a secure sense of left and right. For example, confronted with the figure 13, they may be unsure whether the 3 or the 1 should be considered first and therefore may wonder if the number should be thought of as 'thirteen' or as 'thirty-one'; or again, if required to do long multiplication, they may show hesitation as to whether to work from left to right or from right to left. In addition they may fail to do themselves justice in arithmetic tests because of difficulties or uncertainty in reading the instructions. In the case of these children, however, one hesitates to say that they have a *special* difficulty in arithmetic over and above the difficulties which constitute their dyslexia.

To other dyslexic children, however, arithmetic presents special extra problems. They cannot do subtraction, except of a very simple kind, unless they somehow provide for themselves a visible or tangible representation of the numbers involved; they may need, for instance, to count on their figures, to put marks on paper, or to use bricks or beads if they are to operate with numbers at all. In many cases, too, they have quite remarkable difficulty in memorising arithmetical tables. These, it seems, are special handicaps additional to those regularly associated with dyslexia.

We shall begin this chapter with some suggestions designed to help the majority of dyslexic children over arithmetic; we shall then consider possible ways of helping those (perhaps a minority) for whom arithmetic presents these special additional problems.

One obvious way of helping dyslexic children over arithmetic is to try to improve their sense of left-right awareness. By the time that they come to you it is likely that they will already have worked out a number of compensating devices for themselves or been shown them by their parents, e.g. 'I know it is my *right* hand because I *write* with it' (though you should remember that this pun will not help left-handers), 'My left hand is the one with my watch on', or even, where appropriate, 'My left hand is the one where there is the small scar'. These devices should certainly be encouraged, as should any kind of activity which helps them to appreciate that writing movements should be in the direction that we call 'left to right'. They may, of course, be confused over the *words* 'left' and 'right' quite apart from being unsure which way to move or point. We have met children who, when given the instruction, 'Point to my right eye (or ear) with your left hand', have *consistently* pointed to the tester's left and when asked to point to his left eye or ear have *consistently* pointed to his right. One needs to check, therefore, both whether they can do the right thing and whether they can use the right word.

Let us take a particular example. To a young dyslexic child the signs $>$ and $<$ ('greater than' and 'less than') are easily confused. We suggest that when he needs to read them he should *write them first*. Having written one of the two lines, he should *go back to the beginning* before starting the other. Thus he should not write the lines like this

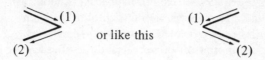

or like this

since in that case it is less easy to tell the difference between them. On the contrary, his movements should be like this,

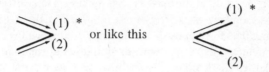

or like this

At the point marked * he should take the pen off and return to his starting-point. From many other situations he will have learned that what we call the 'left' marks the *beginning* of a word. The following rule may then help him: if the beginning is big and moves to something small, the sign means 'greater than'; if the beginning is small and moves to something big, the sign means 'less than'.

For most dyslexic children anything which gives them a firmer sense of left and right is likely to prevent errors in arithmetic.

We shall now consider the needs of those dyslexic children for whom arithmetic presents special extra problems. These are children who, although sometimes quite capable of grasping very sophisticated mathematical notions, display the difficulties described on p. 52: they cannot subtract without special aids, e.g. using their fingers, and they find it very difficult to memorise arithmetical tables.

We are not suggesting, of course, that all children who require such 'aids' are necessarily dyslexic. Just as a five- or six-year-old may put the letter *s* the wrong way round or make other directional mistakes without being dyslexic, so some younger children may be helped by using their fingers for subtraction, and indeed may continue to do so even at age nine or ten when in fact they could manage without. In our experience, however, some older dyslexic children are *dependent* on using their fingers or other aids. Where this happens it should clearly be regarded as a limitation, just as their difficulty over spelling represents a limitation; it can be compensated for but not removed.

How, then, can those with these special difficulties best be helped?

One of the first things is that both teacher and pupil should recognise their existence. They are no accident but part of the total dyslexia picture. This becomes obvious, for instance, the moment one tries to teach arithmetical tables to a dyslexic child; it is not that he happens not to have learned them, but rather that he has certain difficulties in memorising which have *prevented* him from learning them. Similarly the difficulties which some dyslexic children experience over subtraction are completely at variance with their mathematical ability in other ways, just as their difficulties over spelling are at variance with their ability at complex reasoning tasks.

The next point is to make clear to the child that mathematics is something quite different from calculation. It is therefore particularly important that he should not suppose he is 'no good at maths' just because difficulties over calculation are holding him back. It is not enough, however, merely to tell him this. What is needed is experience of success; he needs to find out for himself that he can grasp complicated mathematical ideas. We know of one person who was severely dyslexic and could not even do subtraction sums without using his fingers; yet he acquired enough knowledge of mathematical principles to become a university lecturer in physics. We have also met many boys with similar limitations who have been keen and interested enough to attempt mathematics at O and even A level. Difficulties over calculation are a nuisance, but for those with an aptitude for mathematics they need not be an insurmountable obstacle.

Similar encouragement can sometimes be given to a dyslexic child who is keen on music. Our evidence in this area is limited, but we have come across several children whose dyslexia made sight-reading from a stave difficult, but who nevertheless were extremely gifted musically. It seems likely in these cases that they will learn eventually to read music, just as they learn to read books; but the musical stave has much of the complexity of the printed word and they are therefore likely to experience considerable difficulty with it in the early stages.

54

Ability to cope quickly with conventional musical notation, however, is quite a different thing from ability to appreciate music, and it seems important that they should be aware of this.

We shall now make some suggestions on how best to help a child who needs aids (such as his fingers, marks on paper, or bricks or beads) in order to do calculations. It is very unwise, in our view, to suggest to him that such aids are inherently undesirable. What he needs to realise are their drawbacks, viz. that they take extra time and that their use involves considerable risk of error. For example, if a child can recognise instantaneously that seven from nineteen is twelve, he can proceed immediately to the next part of the problem; if, on the other hand, he has to make nineteen marks on paper, cross seven of them off, and count up the remainder, this takes valuable time and there is serious danger that at some stage he may count wrongly.

If some new mathematical idea is being introduced, it is important that he should not at the same time be troubled with problems of computation. For example, if the intention is to teach him that to obtain area one multiplies length by breadth, one can tell him that if the length is 7 m and the breadth 8 m the area will be 7 x 8 sq.m, but it is a tiresome distraction if he then has to spend time considering what 7 x 8 is! This is no place to discuss the merits of so-called modern mathematics; what is quite clear, in our opinion, is that whatever type of mathematics is taught to a dyslexic child his limitations need to be taken into account. Just as in free composition he can be encouraged to concentrate on what he writes, not on its spelling, so in certain kinds of mathematics he can be encouraged to concentrate on the mathematical ideas involved and not on the computation.

Finally, let us consider the special needs of those dyslexic children who have difficulty with arithmetical tables.

The following are some of the main things which we have noticed in the last few years.

i   Where there is some obvious rule, the child is able to apply it; if he is asked, for example, what is a certain number multiplied by ten, he can usually give the right answer. If, however, he relies on 'just remembering', he is likely to have difficulty with the more awkward tables; thus one would be surprised if 'off the cuff' he could respond correctly to 'What is seven times nine?'

ii   If asked to 'recite' tables in the traditional way (e.g. '1 x 2 = 2,

2 x 2 = 4' etc.) he may be able to cope with the 2, 3, and 4 times tables simply by adding as he goes along, and the 5 times is unlikely to present difficulty. Beyond this, however, he is particularly liable to lose his place. Thus, after reciting the 6 times table correctly up to, say, 5 x 6 = 30, he may need to repeat '5 x 6 = 30' a second or third time (to anchor himself, as it were), or he may suddenly pass to '7 x 6', or perhaps pause and say to the tester, 'Where have I got to?'

iii Some children can overcome this difficulty if they speak extra fast, and some of the brighter ones, when asked to say their 6 times table, will simply say 'six, twelve, eighteen' etc. as fast as they can. If they are then asked to go slowly and to say '1 x 6 = 6, 2 x 6 = 12', etc., the difficulties described under **ii** reappear.

We regard it as quite unnecessary to expect dyslexic children to *recite* tables in this way. What they need is to be able to *operate* with figures when they are required to multiply and divide. It does not matter at all, for example, if they lose their place saying the 8 times table, but it *does* matter if they need to do a calculation and cannot easily decide what is 8 x 7.

Where small numbers are involved, e.g. 2 x 3, no special compensatory devices are necessary. It is likely, presumably as a result of familiarity, that most dyslexic children will simply *remember* that 2 x 3 = 6, and even if they do not they can easily make three pairs of marks on the paper and count them up. In the case of larger numbers, however, e.g. 8 x 7, the product will be both difficult to remember and difficult to calculate. We are not saying that it is flatly impossible for a dyslexic child to learn the answers to multiplication tables by heart, but at best it will take a long time; and the teacher may therefore prefer to rely instead on the slide-rule and the table-square.

We have met a number of older boys who said that they had found the slide-rule a special help, and there is perhaps a case, if a child is dyslexic, for introducing it at a relatively early age, perhaps at eleven or twelve.

At an even earlier age one can introduce the table-square. This is simply a sheet of paper with the digits 1 – 12 running both across and downwards.

Most children, when they understand what is needed, will be able to complete the easy parts of this table-square for themselves. Here is one

in which the 2 times, 3 times, 5 times, 10 times and part of the 11
times have been filled in:

1	2	3	4	5	6	7	8	9	10	11	12
2	4	6	8	10	12	14	16	18	20	22	24
3	6	9	12	15	18	21	24	27	30	33	36
4	8	12		20					40	44	
5	10	15	20	25	30	35	40	45	50	55	60
6	12	18		30					60	66	
7	14	21		35					70	77	
8	16	24		40					80	88	
9	18	27		45					90	99	
10	20	30	40	50	60	70	80	90	100	110	120
11	22	33	44	55	66	77	88	99	110		
12	24	36		60					120		

In due course the rest can be completed, if necessary with the teacher's
help; and if the child needs to find out, for instance, what is 8 x 7, he
simply has to look across to the point where the appropriate row meets
the appropriate column and read off the answer. No memorising or
calculation are called for.

The 5 times, 10 times, and 11 times table follow obvious rules
which can be explained to the child as necessary. Perhaps, however, it is
worth quoting the less well-known rules which help with the 6 times and
9 times. If you are multiplying an even number by 6, the first figure will
be half that number, while the second figure will be the number itself.
(This is because an even number times 5 must end in 0 and there is then
the even number itself to add). In the case of all numbers in the 9 times
table (except 99) the two digits add up to 9. The rule here is: to
multiply a number by nine, subtract *one* from that number; this will be
the first digit, while the second added to the first will make the total
come to 9. Another way of multiplying by 9 is to use the 10 times table
as a kind of 'anchor'. In that case, to multiply a number by 9 one can
multiply it by 10 and then subtract the number. It can be explained that
in arithmetic there may be different ways of arriving at the correct
answer, and that for a dyslexic child the standard, quick method is not
necessarily the right one.

More help for dyslexic children

From what has been said it is plain that an examination involving mathematics could be quite an ordeal for those dyslexic children who experience the difficulties which we have described. One boy reported that he had wasted about three-quarters of an hour in an A level examination through misreading the direction sign ($<$) on a vector line (cf. the difficulties over 'greater than' and 'less than' mentioned above, pp. 52-53. He had realised that his answer must be wrong but could not understand why. In the case of those who can work only with the aids which we have described (their fingers, etc.), there is danger of errors in calculation, and extra time is therefore needed for checking. A sympathetic Examining Board seems essential (and our limited evidence suggests that in fact many Examining Boards take the problems of the dyslexic candidate seriously); and teachers and parents can help on the morale side by encouraging the child to take his time and not to panic. Some preliminary practice at doing arithmetical calculations under pressure of time may serve to acclimatise him to the examination atmosphere.

Our general conclusion is that difficulties over calculation can be a nuisance, but that they need not be an insuperable obstacle to the learning of mathematics. Here, as in other areas, it is perfectly possible for a person with dyslexia to achieve success.

APPENDIX

Section I Consonants for recognition*

a *Words for checking recognition of initial consonant
(also 'x' at the end of a word)*

p and b		c and g		m and n	
pat	bat	can	gun	met	net
pen	bed	cot	got	map	nap
pig	big	cap	gap	mug	nut
pop	bun	cut	get	men	neck

* Suggestions as to how to use the word-lists in this section are given on pp. 21-24. For rules which indicate when to put -*tch* instead of -*ch* and when to put -*ck* instead of -*k* see also p. 28-29.

58

t and d		f and v		w	x	y	z
tip	dip	fan	van	web	box	yes	zip
tap	Dad	fed	vest	win	mix	yell	zigzag
ten	deck	fit	vet	will	six		
tick	dig	fog			next		

b *Words for checking recognition of two consonants*
(one sound heard)

th	sh and ch		qu	wh
this	shut	chat	quiz	when
them	ship	chip	quack	which
thick	shed	chest	quick	whisk
thank	shop	chop		

c *Words for checking recognition of*
two consonants (both sounds heard)

sc/sk	sl	sm	sn	sp	st	sw
scab	slip	smash	snip	spit	step	swim
skin	slug	smell	snack	spot	stand	swing

br	cr	dr	fr	gr	pr	tr
brick	crab	drum	frost	grab	pram	trot
bring	crust	drink	fresh	grit	prick	trust

bl	cl	fl	gl	pl	tw
black	clap	flag	glad	plan	twin
blot	clock	flick	glum	plum	twig

Since 'th' and 'sh' should be thought of as a single unit we may add:

thr	shr
thrush	shrink
thrill	shrub

d *Words for checking recognition of*
   three consonants (all sounds heard)

scr	spr	str	spl
scrub	spring	strap	split
scratch	sprung	stretch	splash

e *Words for checking recognition of final consonants*

-ff	-ss	-zz	-ll	-ng	-nk
cuff	miss	fizz	bell	bang	ink
stiff	dress	buzz	doll	sing	tank

-nd	-nch	-ft	-ct	-mp	-lk
and	pinch	left	fact	pump	milk
pond	lunch	gift	insect	limp	silk

Section II More vowel sounds*

-ue and -ew				-au and -aw		
cue	residue	few	screw	Paul	nau*gh*ty	saw
due	virtue	new	yew	haul	hau*gh*ty	paw
true	issue	chew	view	sauce	dau*gh*ter	law
glue	tissue	grew	phew!	saucer	slau*gh*ter	raw
blue		blew		cause	haunt	jaw
Tuesday		threw		because	gaunt	gnaw
value		*k*new		August	launch	thaw
argue		slew		autumn	laundry	straw
continue		drew		cau*gh*t	caution	lawn
rescue		stew		tau*gh*t		yawn
avenue		crew				sawn
						awful

* These vowel sounds are additional to those given in *On helping the dyslexic child*. Suggestions as to how they should be used are given on p. 25. Where a consonant or pair of consonants is silent (such as the *gh* in *weight*) the silent letters have been italicised to enable them to be picked out more easily.

-ey and -ei

they	their	eight
grey	heir	weight
convey	vein	sleigh
survey	veil	neigh
obey	rein	neighbour
		reign

-ie and -ei (with 'c')

thief	piece	ceiling
chief	niece	conceit
grief	shriek	deceit
brief	yield	receive
belief	wield	perceive
relief	shield	conceive
handkerchief	grieve	
	achieve	

-ow (long 'o')

bow (violin)
bow (tie)
sow (seed)
mow
row (boat)
row (line)
tow (pull)
know
flow
show
snow
grow
throw
follow
swallow
furrow
arrow
bellow

e-e

Peter	impede	scene
meter	concede	intervene
these	theme	athlete
eve	scheme	complete
swede	extreme	concrete
stampede	supreme	obsolete
centipede	serene	

Vowel sounds with additional 'r'

ai + 4 and a-e + r †

fair (colour)	fare (bus)
fair (swings)	bare (uncovered)
pair (two)	dare
hair (on head)	hare (animal)
stairs (steps)	stare (look hard)
chair	rare
	mare
	share
	scare
	spare

oa + r and o-e + r

oar (of boat)	ore (mineral)
boar (animal)	bore (make a hole)
roar	bore (tedious person)
soar (rise)	sore (painful)
	more
	tore
	wore
	core
	shore
	score
	snore
	store

ea + r

dear (darling)
dear (expensive)
ear
fear
gear
hear
near
rear
clear
spear
shears
appear

ee + r

deer (animal)
beer
jeer
cheer
peer
steer
veer
queer

e-e + r

here
mere
sphere
severe
austere
interfere
adhere

† Some words having this sound are spelled -ear, in particular *bear*, *pear*, *tear*, *wear* and *swear*.

Section III Single and double consonants in the middle of a word *

Double consonant (short vowel)	Single consonant (long vowel)
kipper	wiper
hopping	hoping
saddle	cradle
little	title
fiddle	bridle
potted	voted
jazzy	lazy
Jimmy	slimy
bonny	bony

hobble	noble
dinner	finer
sitting	biting
snuggle	bugle
better	Peter
dabble	table
nibble	bible
tabby	baby

* For the rule explaining whether to put a single or a double consonant see p. 28.

Section IV Word-endings

Group A *Words ending in -ey* *

honey	barley
money	parsley
donkey	journey
monkey	chimney
hockey	kidney
jockey	abbey
valley	turkey (Turkey)
volley	jersey (Jersey)
pulley	Guernsey
trolley	Anglesey

Group B *Words in -le and el* †

-le	-el
table	parcel
uncle	Rachel
buckle	satchel
saddle	angel
rifle	parallel
gargle	camel
ripple	panel
little	barrel
muscle	mackerel
castle	easel
bristle	tinsel
whistle	vessel
dazzle	novel
	towel
	hazel
	cruel

* For discussion see p. 36.
† For discussion see p. 37 seq.

Exceptions:

measles (-le instead of -el); and *label, rebel* (noun), *model, chapel, gospel,* and *hostel* (-el instead of -le).

Common words in -ible

terrible	sensible	(ir)responsible
horrible	(in)edible	convertible
(im)possible	(in)audible	collapsible
	(in)visible	eligible
	(il)legible	accessible
	(un)intelligible	

Group C *Words in -ture* ‡

nature	mixture
creature	fracture
picture	puncture
lecture	scripture
future	furniture
capture	temperature

Group D *Words in -cion, -shion, -tion, -sion, and -ssion* *

-cion	-shion
suspicion	cushion
coercion	fashion

-tion after 'n' and 'r'

mention	portion
attention	proportion
detention	exertion
invention	insertion
prevention	assertion
intervention	desertion
	extortion
	distortion
	abortion

-sion after 'n' and 'r'

pension	version
tension	diversion
dimension	conversion
extension	aversion
mansion	submersion
expansion	immersion
apprehension	excursion

‡ For discussion see p. 40.
* For discussion see pp. 42-43 seq.

-ssion

confession	session	mission	depression	discussion
profession	possession	admission	oppression	concussion
	accession	omission	expression	percussion
	succession	submission	impression	repercussion
	procession	permission		
	aggression	commission		
		transmission		

Group E *Words in -age, -ace, and -ate †*

-age	-ace	-ate
cabbage	preface	certificate
bandage	surface	delicate
baggage	palace	duplicate
luggage	furnace	intricate
package	terrace	frigate
village		intermediate
image		appropriate
manage		desolate
cottage		disconsolate
voyage		consulate
drainage		climate
coinage		senate
average		subordinate
encourage		
passage		
advantage		
shortage		
postage		
savage		
marriage ‡		
carriage ‡		

† For discussion see pp. 43-44.
‡ the *i* in these words is not heard.

Group F *Adjectives ending in -ous* *

a *Adjectives with a consonant or 'ge' before the -ous*

famous	gorgeous	tremendous
joyous	generous	courageous
nervous	poisonous	adventurous
pompous	prosperous	monotonous

b *Adjectives ending in -ious or -eous*

obvious	courteous
various	hideous
serious	erroneous
curious	spontaneous
furious	simultaneous
envious	instantaneous
glorious	
previous	
bilious	
copious	
harmonious	
melodious	
religious †	
contagious †	

c *Adjectives with either -ci- or -ti- followed by -ous, and also
-sci- and -xi- followed by -ous*

-tious	-cious	-scious	-xious
ambitious	gracious	conscious	anxious
cautious	precious	unconscious	noxious
pretentious	delicious		
licentious	suspicious		
infectious	vicious		
	ferocious		
	atrocious		
	precocious		
	officious		
	capacious		

* For discussion see p. 44.
† The *i* in these words is not heard.

Group G *Words in -al* ‡

Nouns in -al which can be adjectives		**Other nouns in -al**

Nouns in -al which can be adjectives		Other nouns in -al
general	serial	sandal
corporal	material	rascal
principal	moral	dial
liberal	diagonal	phial
cannibal	cathedral	coral
mortal	terminal	vandal
animal	aerial	cymbal
pedal		jackal
signal		medal
mineral		pedestal
funeral		interval
		hospital

Adjectives in -tial and -cial

-tial	**-cial**	
spatial	facial	beneficial
initial	racial	superficial
partial	special	social
essential *	judicial	commercial
	official	crucial
	financial *	
	provincial *	

‡ For discussion see pp. 44-46.

* All adjectives with *n* before the 'shŭl' -ending are spelled -tial, except *financial* and *provincial*.

Group H *Common words in -ent and -ant †*

-ent		-ant	
Nouns	*Adjectives*	*Nouns*	*Adjectives*
resident	confident	descendant	abundant
student	evident	attendant	radiant
client	independent	infant	defiant
opponent	impudent	merchant	brilliant
serpent	obedient	elephant	luxuriant
parent	convenient	giant	vigilant
gradient	silent	tenant	gallant ‡
talent	excellent	informant	indignant ‡
Orient	violent	assailant	dominant
continent	insolent	participant	fragrant
accident	permanent	peasant	pleasant
current (water	prominent	pheasant	distant
or electricity)	apparent ‡	inhabitant	instant
	different	consultant	relevant
	absent	contestant	observant
	consistent	assistant	
	frequent	truant	
	eloquent	currant (fruit)	

Note.   All adjectives have corresponding nouns ending in *-ance* and
-ence except those marked ‡

† For discussion see p. 47.

Section V   Sentences for practice of words in groups D and F of section IV

1 I have a suspicion that the government may decide to use coercion.
2 Cushions are out of fashion.
3 You can read the shorter version of the story on your excursion.

* For discussion see pp. 35, 36, 43 and 44 and Appendix, Section IV (Groups
D and F), pp. 65 and 67.

  4 The mansion has no room for extension or expansion.

  5 Can he afford an immersion heater if he is on a pension?

  6 From the discussion at the morning session I had the impression that there was no charge for admission.

  7 In his confession he said that he had been in possession of a car without the owner's permission.

  8 The floats in the procession came in quick succession.

  9 After the explosion everyone was feeling the tension, but there was no occasion for apprehension.

10 The mention of a new invention at once attracted his attention.

11 He never failed to be generous even after he had become prosperous.

12 How courageous of you to speak when you felt so nervous!

13 Previously he had never been serious about his religious beliefs.

14 The two events were simultaneous.

15 He admitted quite spontaneously that his statement had been erroneous.

16 The school had to be cautious in case the illness was infectious.

17 I am anxious in case the noxious fumes make him unconscious before help comes.

18 I am always suspicious of anyone who acts in an officious manner.

19 The animal was vicious and had a ferocious bark.

20 Her spelling is atrocious but her cooking is delicious.

References

A large number of books have recently been published on the subject of dyslexia. In our experience, however, long book lists are somewhat daunting, and rather than try to draw up a comprehensive review of the literature it seemed to us that it would be more helpful simply to mention a few of these books (including some already mentioned in *On helping the dyslexic child*) which we thought would help those parents and teachers who wish to do some further reading. With this objective in mind we recommend:

1   M. CRITCHLEY, *The Dyslexic Child*. Heinemann Medical Books, 1971.
2   ALFRED WHITE FRANKLIN and SANDHYA NAIDOO (eds.), *Assessment and Teaching of Dyslexic Children*. Invalid Children's Aid Association, London, 1970.
3   ANNA GILLINGHAM and BESSIE W. STILLMAN, *Remedial Training for Children with Specific Disability in Reading, Spelling and Penmanship*. Cambridge, Massachusets, 1956.
4   K. HERMANN, *Reading Disability*. Munksgaard, Copenhagen, 1959.
5   S. NAIDOO, *Specific Dyslexia*. Pitman, 1972.
6   M.D. VERNON, *Reading and Its Difficulties*. Cambridge, 1971.

The following books are mentioned in Chapter I as being of historical interest:

7   J. HINSHELWOOD, *Letter-, Word-, and Mind-Blindness*. H.K. Lewis, 1900.
8   J. HINSHELWOOD, *Congenital Word-Blindness*. H.K. Lewis, 1917.
9   M. MACMEEKEN. *Ocular Dominance in Relation to Developmental Aphasia*. University of London Press, 1939.
10 S.T. ORTON, *Reading, Writing and Speech Problems in Children*. Chapman and Hall, 1937.

There are two more reference books which we should like to mention. They are:

11   E.L. THORNDIKE and I. LORGE, *The Teacher's Word Book of 30,000 Words.* New York, 1944.
12   LAWRENCE H. DAWSON, *Walker's Rhyming Dictionary of the English Language.* Routledge and Kegan Paul, 1924.

Those who wish to discover the frequency of occurrence of any word in the English language will find some helpful information in 11, while 12, which arranges words alphabetically in inverse order of their letters, may be of use to those wishing to do further work on word-endings.

Index

-able (word-ending)   38, 39
-ace (word-ending)   43, 66
ad- (word-beginning)   50
-age (word-ending)   43, 66
-al (word-ending)   44, 68
A level, see under 'examinations'
-ance (word-ending)   69
Anderson, J.   17
-ant (word-ending)   47, 69
aphasia   3
-ary (word-ending)   46
-ate (word-ending)   43, 66

brain damage   3
British Dyslexia Association   4

ch and *tch* rule   28, 29, 32
Chaplin, M.B.   17
Chronically Sick and Disabled
      Persons Act   4
-cion (word-ending)   43, 65
circum- (word-beginning)   48
ck and *k* rule   v, 28, 29
con- (word-beginning)   48
CSE, see under 'examinations'
Critchley, M.   71

Daniels, J.C.   17
Dawson, L.M.   72
de- (word-beginning)   49
developmental aphasia   1
Diack, H.   17
dictionary, training in use of
      26, 27
directional confusion   2, see also
      under 'spatial confusion'
dis- (word-beginning)   49

doubling-the-consonant rule   v,
      28
dys- (word-beginning)   50

-ed (word-ending)   37
-el (word-ending)   37, 64
en- (word-beginning)   49
-ence (word-ending)   47, 69
-ent (word-ending)   47, 69
-er (word-ending)   37
-ery (word-ending)   46
examinations   4, 10, 11, 42, 54,
      58
-ey (word-ending)   36, 64

family relationships   9
Franklin, A.W.   3, 71

Garratt, C.   v
Gillingham, A.   2, 71
greater than/less than,   52, 53
Grice, F.   71

hard/soft *c* and *g* rule   28
hard/soft consonants   38
Hermann, K.   71
Hinshelwood, J.   2, 71

in- (word-beginning)   49
-ible (word-ending)   38, 39, 65
in- (word-beginning)   49
-ing (word-ending)   36
inter- (word-beginning)   48
Invalid Children's Aid Association
      3

Ladybird Key Words Reading
      Scheme   18

-le (word-ending)   37, 64
look and say' teaching method   17, 18
Lorge, I.   72
-ly (word-ending)   36

MacMeeken, H.   2, 71
McCullagh, S.K.   17
marker, use of   15, 16
Miles, J.E.   17
mis- (word-beginning)   48
Murray, W.   18
music, reading of   54

Naidoo, S.   3, 71

O level, see under 'examinations'
Orton Society   2
Orton S.T.   2, 71
-ous (word-ending)   44, 67

per- (word-beginning)   48
phonic approach   iv, 17, 18
pre- (word-beginning)   49
pro- (word-beginning)   49
psychiatric help   2, 11

re- (word-beginning)   49
repetition, use of   1
reporter's note book, use of   25, 26

-s (word-ending)   39
'same-different' technique   22
Schonell, F.J.   17
Scott, Sir Walter   6

-shion (word-ending)   43, 65
-sion (word-ending)   43, 65
slide rule, use of   56
social relationships   9
spatial confusion   1, 51, 52, 53
specific developmental dyslexia   1
specific language disability   1
-ssion (word-ending)   43, 66
Stillman, B.W.   2, 71
Stirling, E.   v
strephosymbolia   1, 2
sub- (word-beginning)   50

table square, use of   57
temporal confusion   1, 8
Thatcher, M.   4
Thorndike, E.L.   72
-tion (word-ending)   39, 65
Tizard, J.   4
-ture (word-ending)   40, 65
typewriter, use of   33, 34

Vernon, M.D.   71

Waddon, A.   v
Wiggin, A.V.   v
Word Blind Centre   3
word-blindness   1
writing patterns   18, 19, 20, 21

-y (word-ending)   36

-z (word-ending)   39